OSTEOPOROSIS DIET COOKBOOK FOR SENIORS

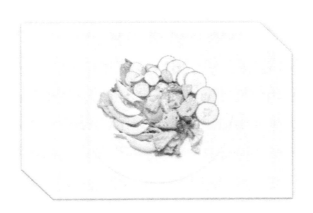

A Comprehensive Guide to Natural Nutrition and Easy Calcium-Rich Recipes for Seniors with Osteoporosis

Dr. Grace Whitfield

Text Copyright© 2025 by Dr. Grace Whitfield

DISCLAIMER

The information provided in this cookbook is for educational purposes only and is not intended as a substitute for professional medical advice, diagnosis, or treatment. While the recipes and dietary guidance in this book are designed to support seniors managing osteoporosis, each individual's health condition and dietary needs are unique.

It is crucial to consult with a healthcare provider or registered dietitian who specializes in bone health before making significant changes to your diet, especially if you have existing medical conditions, are taking medications, or have been given specific dietary recommendations related to your condition.

The author and publisher disclaim any liability for adverse effects or consequences resulting from the use or interpretation of the content in this cookbook. Always seek personalized medical advice to ensure that the dietary choices you make are appropriate for your individual health needs and circumstances.

A NOTE OF GRATITUDE

Dear Reader

Thank you for choosing the *Osteoporosis Diet Cookbook for Seniors*. It is truly an honor to be part of your journey toward stronger bones and improved health. As someone who has worked closely with individuals managing osteoporosis, I deeply understand the challenges that come with maintaining bone health as we age. It is my heartfelt wish that the nutrition guides, meal plans, and recipes in this book will empower you to take control of your health and enhance your quality of life every day.

Remember, small changes in your diet can lead to significant improvements in your bone health, and you are not alone in this journey. May the tools, tips, and recipes in this book inspire you to make informed, nourishing choices that support strong, healthy bones.

Wishing you strength, vitality, and enduring health on your path to a stronger you!

Dr. Grace Whitfield.

This cookbook belongs to:

_____

_____

_____

_____

ABOUT THE AUTHOR

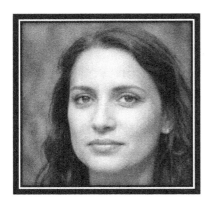 Dr. Grace Whitfield is a nutrition expert with over 15 years of experience in health. She holds a bachelor's degree in nutritional science and a master's degree in gerontology and nutrition. Dr. Grace has collaborated with healthcare providers, caregivers, and community organizations to create personalized dietary plans for individuals managing various chronic conditions such as kidney disease, diabetes, hypertension, and more. She has also worked as a nutritional consultant in diverse care settings, ensuring that clinical requirements are met while also considering clients' preferences for tasty, enjoyable meals. Her cookbooks feature easy-to-prepare, budget-friendly recipes designed to meet a wide range of dietary needs. Dr. Grace's mission is to help individuals of all ages live vibrant, healthy lives through better nutrition.

"Your health is your greatest wealth—invest in it daily."

CONTENTS

Who this cookbook is for

This cookbook is specially designed for seniors managing osteoporosis who are looking for simple, nutritious, and bone-strengthening recipes to support their bone health.

It's for:

- Those who want to take control of their diet while managing osteoporosis.

- Individuals seeking easy-to-follow, calcium-rich recipes tailored to promote bone health.

- Caregivers and family members preparing meals for loved ones with osteoporosis.

If you're ready to enjoy delicious meals that support strong bones and a healthy lifestyle, this cookbook is here to guide you every step of the way!

How to Use This Book

This cookbook is designed to make managing osteoporosis easier and more enjoyable by providing bone-healthy, nutrient-rich recipes. Here's how to get the most out of it:

1. **Understand Your Nutritional Needs**
   Consult your healthcare provider or dietitian to confirm your specific dietary requirements, such as calcium, vitamin D, protein, and magnesium intake. Knowing your personalized needs will help guide your recipe choices.

2. **Choose Recipes That Support Bone Health**
   Each recipe includes ingredient lists and preparation steps focused on strengthening bones. Select meals that align with your health goals and taste preferences while ensuring they meet your nutritional needs.

3. **Plan Ahead**

   Use the recipes to create a weekly meal plan, which will help you stay organized and consistently meet your dietary needs for bone health.

4. **Adjust as Needed**

   Everyone's dietary needs are unique. Feel free to adjust portion sizes or ingredients based on your medical advice or personal preferences, such as incorporating additional calcium or reducing sodium as recommended by your healthcare provider.

5. **Enjoy the Process**

   Eating well to support bone health doesn't have to be restrictive. Experiment with the recipes, enjoy the flavors, and find joy in nourishing your body with foods that promote strong, healthy bones.

With this book as your guide, you can take charge of your bone health while still enjoying satisfying, delicious meals. Here's to your strength, vitality, and well-being!

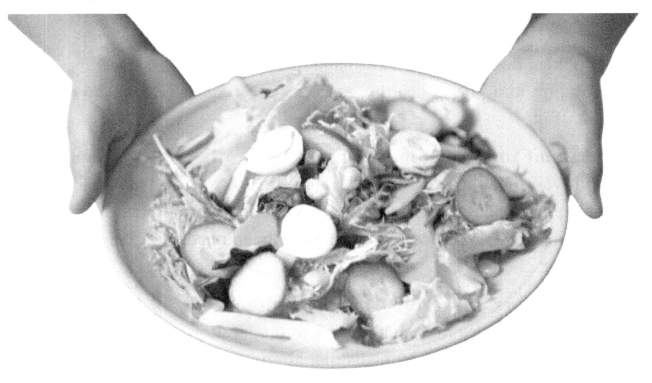

INTRODUCTION

A few years ago, my sister Olivia faced a life-changing diagnosis: osteoporosis. Like many individuals confronted with this condition, she was filled with concern about her future—worried about the potential loss of mobility, independence, and overall quality of life. As a nutritionist with years of experience, I knew we had options beyond the standard treatments. I believed that through a targeted, nutrient-rich diet, we could help her body heal and rebuild naturally.

With careful planning and consistent effort, we made changes to her daily meals—incorporating foods rich in essential nutrients that are critical for bone health. Over time, we saw remarkable progress.

Her bone density stabilized, her energy levels improved, and she started feeling more confident and in control of her health. What Olivia and I discovered through this journey is something I have always known in theory but saw confirmed in practice: nutrition has the power to transform health, particularly when it comes to conditions like osteoporosis.

Olivia's success inspired me to create this book, **The Osteoporosis Diet Cookbook for Seniors**. It's my mission to share the strategies that worked for her with a broader audience—people like you, who may be facing the same challenges, looking for natural, sustainable ways to manage and improve your bone health.

Whether you've just been diagnosed with osteoporosis, or you're seeking preventive measures to protect your bones, this cookbook is designed to be your trusted guide.

In this book, you will find carefully crafted recipes that emphasize foods rich in nutrients that promote bone density and strength. These are not just random recipes—they are specifically designed to nourish your body in ways that support strong bones, reduce the risk of fractures, and help slow down or even reverse the progression of osteoporosis. You'll find a wide variety of meals that are both simple to prepare and delicious to enjoy, from breakfasts that energize your day to dinners that nourish your body deeply.

But this book isn't just about what's on your plate—it's about empowerment.

By choosing the right foods, you are taking control of your health in a proactive, natural way. I've seen the power of this approach firsthand, both in my sister's journey and in the countless patients I've worked with over the years. I want you to experience the same transformation.

Each recipe in this cookbook is backed by nutritional science and is built around ingredients that are readily available, so you can easily incorporate them into your daily routine. And because I know how challenging it can be to stick to a dietary plan, I've made sure that these meals are not only nutritious but also enjoyable, making it easier for you to stay on track.

The path to stronger bones and better health is possible, and it starts with the food you eat.

Through the recipes in this book, I'll guide you toward dietary changes that can truly make a difference. Whether you're cooking for yourself or a loved one, these recipes will help support your bone health journey in a natural and sustainable way.

I'm thrilled to have the opportunity to share my knowledge and passion with you through **The Osteoporosis Diet Cookbook for Seniors**. Let's begin this journey toward stronger bones and a healthier, more vibrant future—one meal at a time.

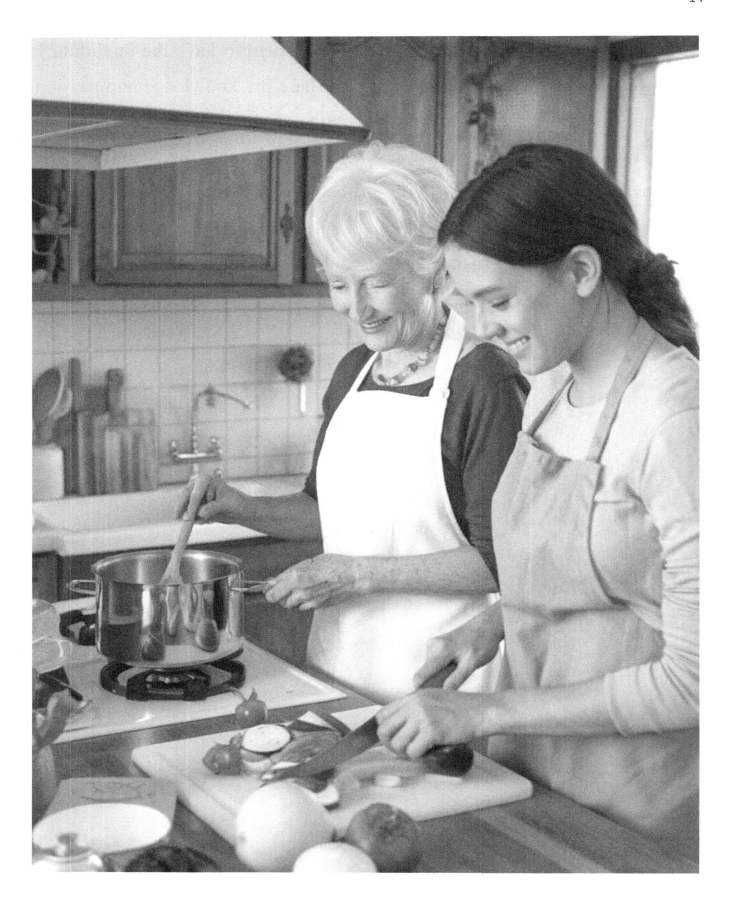

CHAPTER: 1

Osteoporosis: A Comprehensive Overview

Osteoporosis is a chronic, progressive condition characterized by a decrease in bone mass and density, which leads to fragile bones and an increased risk of fractures. Known as a **"silent disease"** because it progresses without symptoms until a fracture occurs, osteoporosis is a significant health concern worldwide, particularly for seniors. In this comprehensive explanation, we will explore what osteoporosis is, why it is of special concern for seniors, its causes, symptoms, and preventive measures that can help reduce its impact.

What is Osteoporosis?

Osteoporosis, derived from the Greek words for **"porous bones,"** is a medical condition where bones become weak, brittle, and more susceptible to fractures, often from minor falls or, in severe cases, even simple movements like bending or coughing. Healthy bones are in a constant state of regeneration. Old bone is broken down and replaced with new bone tissue. However, as individuals age, this balance can shift, and the creation of new bone may not keep pace with the removal of old bone, leading to decreased bone density and strength.

Bone density is usually at its peak in a person's 20s or early 30s.

After that, the rate of bone loss begins to exceed the rate of bone formation. Osteoporosis occurs when bone loss becomes so significant that the bone's structure weakens, increasing the risk of fractures. The bones most affected by osteoporosis include the spine, hips, and wrists, although it can impact any part of the skeletal system.

Why Osteoporosis is a Concern for Seniors:

Osteoporosis is particularly concerning for seniors due to the combination of aging and the natural decline in bone density that occurs as people grow older. In fact, according to the National Osteoporosis Foundation (NOF), approximately 54 million Americans have low bone mass or osteoporosis, with women and seniors being at the highest risk. Globally, osteoporosis affects hundreds of millions of people, with older adults representing the largest proportion of this demographic.

There are several reasons why osteoporosis is such a critical health concern for seniors:

1. Higher Risk of Fractures: As bones become more fragile, seniors are at an increased risk of fractures. Hip fractures, in particular, can be devastating, often leading to long-term disability, loss of independence, or even death in severe cases. Wrist and spinal fractures are also common and can significantly impair mobility and quality of life.

2. **Compromised Mobility:** Osteoporosis can limit an individual's ability to perform everyday tasks. Fractures in the spine, for example, can lead to chronic back pain, height loss, and a hunched posture, further restricting movement and causing discomfort.

3. **Complications in Healing:** As we age, the body's ability to heal diminishes. Seniors with osteoporosis face longer recovery times from fractures, and in some cases, the bone may not heal correctly, leading to chronic issues or further deterioration of health.

4. **Increased Healthcare Costs:** Osteoporosis-related fractures contribute to substantial healthcare costs due to hospitalizations, surgeries (like hip replacements), long-term rehabilitation, and the need for assistive care.

5. **Loss of Independence:** For many seniors, the loss of mobility and function due to osteoporosis-related fractures can lead to dependence on caregivers, moving to assisted living facilities, or the need for continuous home care.

What Causes Osteoporosis?

The causes of osteoporosis are multifactorial, involving a combination of genetic, environmental, and lifestyle factors that affect bone density over time. Key factors contributing to the development of osteoporosis include:

1. **Age**: As mentioned, age is the primary risk factor for osteoporosis. Bone density peaks in early adulthood and gradually declines with age. After menopause, women experience a more rapid loss of bone mass due to a significant drop in estrogen, a hormone that helps protect bone strength.

2. **Gender**: Women are more likely than men to develop osteoporosis, particularly after menopause. Estrogen, which plays a crucial role in maintaining bone density, decreases sharply during menopause, leaving postmenopausal women at a much higher risk of osteoporosis.

3. **Family History**: Genetics also play a role in osteoporosis risk. If a person's parents or grandparents had osteoporosis or fractures, especially of the hip, spine, or wrist, their own risk is increased.

4. **Hormonal Imbalances**: Besides estrogen, other hormones such as testosterone in men and thyroid hormones can affect bone density. Excessive thyroid hormone (hyperthyroidism) can lead to bone loss, as can imbalances in parathyroid and adrenal hormones.

5. **Nutritional Deficiencies**: Calcium and vitamin D are critical nutrients for maintaining strong bones. A lifelong lack of adequate calcium intake contributes to diminished bone density, and vitamin D is necessary for the body to absorb calcium.

Deficiencies in these nutrients are common contributors to osteoporosis.

6. **Sedentary Lifestyle:** Physical activity, particularly weight-bearing exercises, is essential for building and maintaining bone strength. Individuals who are inactive or bedridden for extended periods are at higher risk of developing osteoporosis.

7. **Medications:** Long-term use of certain medications, such as corticosteroids (e.g., prednisone), can lead to significant bone loss. Other drugs that may contribute to osteoporosis include certain antiepileptic medications, thyroid hormones, and medications used to treat breast cancer and prostate cancer.

8. **Alcohol and Smoking:** Both smoking and excessive alcohol consumption are known to weaken bones. Smoking impairs the body's ability to absorb calcium, while heavy drinking can interfere with bone formation and increase the risk of falls.

Symptoms of Osteoporosis:

Osteoporosis is often referred to as a "silent disease" because it develops without noticeable symptoms. People may not realize they have osteoporosis until they experience a fracture, which is often the first sign. However, as the condition progresses, certain symptoms may become apparent, including:

1. **Fractures from Minor Injuries:** One of the most common and telling signs of osteoporosis is experiencing fractures from

minor falls or, in severe cases, simple actions like bending over or coughing. Fractures of the wrist, spine, and hip are particularly common.

2. Loss of Height: As osteoporosis affects the vertebrae, it can lead to a gradual loss of height. This occurs because the weakened bones in the spine may compress or collapse, leading to a stooped posture.

3. Back Pain: Compression fractures in the vertebrae can cause severe back pain. The bones in the spine may weaken and collapse, leading to chronic discomfort, changes in posture, and difficulty moving.

4. Stooped Posture: Also known as kyphosis, this forward-curving of the spine occurs when the bones in the spine fracture and compress, resulting in a hunched posture.

5. Bone Weakness: As the disease progresses, bones become more fragile and may break more easily, even with minimal impact.

Because osteoporosis can go undetected for many years, routine screenings (such as bone density tests) are crucial for early detection, especially for individuals at higher risk.

Preventive Measures for Osteoporosis

While osteoporosis cannot always be fully prevented, especially in individuals with genetic predispositions, there are numerous steps that can be taken to reduce the risk of developing osteoporosis or slow its progression.

Preventive measures focus primarily on lifestyle adjustments and nutrition:

1. **Adequate Calcium Intake**: Calcium is the building block of strong bones, and ensuring a sufficient intake throughout life is one of the most effective ways to maintain bone density. For adults, the recommended daily intake of calcium is around 1,000 to 1,200 milligrams, depending on age and gender. Calcium-rich foods include dairy products (milk, yogurt, cheese), leafy green vegetables (kale, broccoli), and fortified foods (certain cereals, orange juice, and plant-based milks).

2. **Vitamin D Supplementation**: Vitamin D is essential for calcium absorption in the body.

   While sunlight is a primary source of vitamin D, many people, particularly seniors, may require supplements to maintain adequate levels.

   Foods rich in vitamin D include fatty fish (salmon, mackerel), egg yolks, and fortified foods. For those with limited sun exposure, a doctor may recommend vitamin D supplements.

3. **Weight-Bearing Exercises**: Regular physical activity, particularly weight-bearing exercises like walking, jogging, dancing, and strength training, is vital for building and maintaining bone strength. Exercise stimulates bone formation and helps preserve bone density as we age.

4. **Avoid Smoking and Limit Alcohol Consumption**: Quitting smoking and moderating alcohol intake are crucial steps in preventing osteoporosis. Smoking impairs calcium absorption, while excessive alcohol can interfere with bone formation and increase the risk of falls.

5. **Fall Prevention**: Since osteoporosis increases the risk of fractures, fall prevention becomes a key aspect of managing the condition, especially in seniors. This includes making homes safer by reducing tripping hazards, improving lighting, using assistive devices (like canes or walkers), and maintaining physical strength and balance through exercises like tai chi or yoga.

6. **Bone Density Testing**: Routine bone density tests (such as DEXA scans) are important for detecting osteoporosis early, especially for those over the age of 50 or with risk factors. Early detection allows for proactive measures to be taken before fractures occur.

7. **Medications for Bone Health**: In some cases, doctors may prescribe medications such as bisphosphonates, hormone replacement therapy, or other bone-strengthening drugs for individuals at high risk of fractures. These medications can help slow bone loss and, in some cases, even increase bone density.

Conclusion

Osteoporosis is a serious health condition that significantly affects the lives of seniors, but it is not an inevitable consequence of aging. By understanding the causes and symptoms of osteoporosis, as well as implementing preventive strategies, you can take proactive steps to protect your bone health and reduce the risk of fractures. Through a combination of adequate nutrition, regular exercise, and healthy lifestyle choices, osteoporosis can be managed effectively, allowing you to maintain your independence, mobility, and quality of life for years to come.

CHAPTER: 2

What are the health benefits of following this diet:

Following a diet specifically designed to combat osteoporosis offers numerous health benefits beyond just improving bone density. Such a diet, rich in essential nutrients like calcium, vitamin D, magnesium, and other key minerals, can contribute to overall health in multiple ways. Below are the core health benefits of adhering to an osteoporosis diet:

1. Improved Bone Health:

The most obvious benefit of an osteoporosis diet is the enhancement of bone health. By focusing on calcium-rich foods, such as dairy products, leafy greens, and fortified options, the body receives the essential nutrients required for bone formation and maintenance. Adequate calcium intake helps slow down bone density loss, and in some cases, it may even increase bone mass.

Key nutrients:

- **Calcium:** Strengthens bones and teeth.

- **Vitamin D:** Enhances calcium absorption in the intestines.

- **Magnesium:** Supports bone structure by converting vitamin D into its active form, which aids in calcium absorption.

2. Reduced Risk of Fractures

A diet rich in bone-strengthening nutrients reduces the likelihood of bone fractures, which is a major concern for individuals with osteoporosis. Nutrient-dense foods help improve bone density and resilience, making bones less prone to breakage.

This can be particularly helpful in preventing hip, spine, and wrist fractures, which are common in osteoporosis patients.

Key nutrients:

- **Vitamin K:** Essential for bone mineralization and reducing the risk of fractures.

- **Protein:** Provides the building blocks for bone tissue, enhancing bone strength.

3. Enhanced Muscle Function

An osteoporosis diet doesn't just focus on bones—it also promotes healthy muscle function. Protein, vitamin D, and other minerals found in such diets help strengthen muscles, which is crucial for supporting and protecting the skeletal system. Strong muscles reduce the likelihood of falls, a major cause of fractures in people with osteoporosis.

Key nutrients:

- **Protein:** Helps in muscle repair and growth, which supports balance and coordination.

- **Magnesium:** Plays a role in muscle contraction and relaxation.

- **Potassium:** Helps prevent muscle weakness by maintaining electrolyte balance.

4. Improved Joint Health

The nutrients present in an osteoporosis-focused diet can also contribute to better joint health. Magnesium, omega-3 fatty acids, and other key nutrients have anti-inflammatory properties, which help reduce joint stiffness and pain.

This is particularly beneficial for older adults who may suffer from both osteoporosis and arthritis or other joint-related issues.

Key nutrients:

- **Omega-3 fatty acids:** Found in fatty fish like salmon and flaxseeds, these healthy fats reduce inflammation and support joint lubrication.

- **Vitamin C:** Promotes collagen production, which supports cartilage health and reduces joint wear and tear.

5. Better Posture and Mobility

As bone health improves through proper nutrition, the likelihood of developing spine-related issues like kyphosis (a hunched back) is reduced. Strong bones and muscles help maintain good posture, allowing for better mobility and quality of life. Nutrients like vitamin D and magnesium contribute to spinal health and overall skeletal structure, reducing the risk of spinal fractures.

Key nutrients:

- **Vitamin D and Calcium:** Support vertebral strength, preventing spine deformities and fractures.

- **Protein and Magnesium:** Aid in muscle strength and flexibility, improving posture and balance.

6. Cardiovascular Health

Many of the foods that are beneficial for bone health are also good for the heart. For example, leafy greens, fatty fish, and nuts contain nutrients that support cardiovascular health. An osteoporosis diet typically limits processed and high-sodium foods, which are known to contribute to heart disease. Therefore, by improving bone health, individuals can also experience reduced blood pressure, lower cholesterol levels, and overall better cardiovascular function.

Key nutrients:

- **Magnesium and Potassium:** Help regulate blood pressure and improve heart health.

- **Omega-3 fatty acids:** Reduce the risk of heart disease by lowering inflammation and improving cholesterol levels.

7. Weight Management

Proper nutrition plays a key role in maintaining a healthy weight. For people with osteoporosis, excess body weight can place additional strain on the bones and joints, increasing the risk of fractures.

On the other hand, being underweight can also weaken bones, making them more prone to breaks. An osteoporosis diet encourages a balanced intake of nutrients and healthy portion control, helping individuals maintain a healthy weight that supports bone strength.

Key nutrients:

- **Fiber:** Found in whole grains, fruits, and vegetables, fiber helps manage weight by promoting a feeling of fullness.

- **Lean proteins and healthy fats:** Support muscle mass while promoting healthy weight maintenance.

8. Improved Immune Function

The nutrients in an osteoporosis diet, particularly vitamins and minerals, help strengthen the immune system.

A strong immune system is essential for reducing the risk of infections and illnesses that can indirectly worsen osteoporosis symptoms by causing inactivity or bed rest, which can lead to further bone weakening.

Key nutrients:

- **Vitamin C:** Supports the immune system by boosting white blood cell production.

- **Zinc:** Aids in immune function and wound healing, important for recovery from fractures.

9. Support for Mental Health

Nutrition has a profound effect on mental health. The right foods not only improve physical well-being but also contribute to mental and emotional stability. An osteoporosis diet that includes nutrient-dense foods can help reduce feelings of depression and anxiety that often accompany chronic illnesses like osteoporosis. Omega-3 fatty acids and vitamin D, in particular, have been linked to better mood regulation.

Key nutrients:

- **Vitamin D:** Known as the "sunshine vitamin," it plays a role in mood stabilization and reducing the risk of depression.

- **Omega-3 fatty acids:** Promote brain health and reduce inflammation that can contribute to mental health disorders.

10. Longevity and Quality of Life

Overall, following an osteoporosis-focused diet can lead to a longer, healthier life. By preventing fractures, improving mobility, and promoting overall health, such a diet enhances both longevity and quality of life. Seniors who manage their osteoporosis effectively through diet can maintain independence, stay active, and enjoy a better standard of living well into their later years.

Key nutrients:

- **Calcium and Vitamin D:** Support bone longevity, reducing the likelihood of life-threatening fractures.

- **Antioxidants (e.g., Vitamin C and E):** Help protect cells from damage, promoting long-term health.

Conclusion

A diet tailored to address osteoporosis has far-reaching benefits that go well beyond bone health. By incorporating essential nutrients that strengthen bones, reduce the risk of fractures, and support overall health, you can enhance your quality of life, mobility, and longevity. Preventive measures through nutrition can also reduce the emotional and financial burdens of managing osteoporosis-related fractures and complications, making it an essential aspect of a comprehensive approach to healthy aging.

Foods to Eat, Limit, and Avoid for Optimal Bone and Joint Health:

Osteoporosis is a condition that weakens bones, making them fragile and more likely to break. Diet plays a critical role in managing osteoporosis and maintaining bone and joint health. By eating nutrient-rich foods, avoiding those that deplete bone density, and making wise dietary choices, individuals with osteoporosis can strengthen their bones and improve overall health. Below, we will explore the foods to eat, limit, and avoid for achieving optimal bone and joint health.

Foods to Eat for Bone and Joint Health

1. **Calcium-Rich Foods** Calcium is the most crucial mineral for bone health. It strengthens bones and helps maintain their structure.

For individuals with osteoporosis, ensuring adequate calcium intake is vital to slow down bone loss and promote bone formation.

Key sources of calcium include:

- Dairy products: Milk, yogurt, and cheese

- Leafy green vegetables: Kale, broccoli, bok choy, and collard greens

- Fortified foods: Calcium-fortified plant-based milks (such as almond or soy milk), cereals, and orange juice

- Fish: Canned salmon and sardines with bones.

2. **Vitamin D-Rich Foods** Vitamin D is essential for calcium absorption. Without enough vitamin D, the body cannot effectively use the calcium from food, leading to weakened bones. Sunlight exposure helps the body produce vitamin D, but food sources are necessary for those with limited sun exposure.

Key sources of vitamin D include:

o Fatty fish: Salmon, mackerel, and tuna

o Egg yolks

o Fortified foods: Fortified milk, orange juice, and cereals

o Mushrooms (particularly those exposed to sunlight)

3. **Magnesium-Rich Foods** Magnesium is another important mineral that supports bone strength by converting vitamin D into its active form, which helps calcium absorption.

Key sources of magnesium include:

o Nuts and seeds: Almonds, sunflower seeds, and flaxseeds

o Leafy green vegetables: Spinach and Swiss chard

o Whole grains: Brown rice, quinoa, and oats

o Legumes: Lentils, black beans, and chickpeas

4. **Protein-Rich Foods** Protein is crucial for bone and muscle health. It helps repair and build tissues, which is essential for maintaining the skeletal structure and supporting muscle function.

Key sources of protein include:

o Lean meats: Chicken, turkey, and lean cuts of beef or pork.

o Fish: Salmon, sardines, and mackerel.

- Plant-based proteins: Tofu, tempeh, and legumes (like beans and lentils).

- Dairy products: Greek yogurt, cottage cheese, and milk.

5. **Omega-3 Fatty Acids** Omega-3 fatty acids, particularly from fish sources, have anti-inflammatory properties that help reduce joint stiffness and pain, benefiting overall joint health.

Key sources of omega-3s include:

- Fatty fish: Salmon, mackerel, and sardines

- Walnuts and flaxseeds

- Chia seeds

6. **Fruits and Vegetables** Fruits and vegetables are rich in antioxidants, vitamins, and minerals that support bone health and reduce inflammation.

They help prevent the oxidative stress that can weaken bones.

Key sources include:

- Citrus fruits (oranges, lemons): Rich in vitamin C, which is essential for collagen production and bone health.

- Berries: Strawberries, blueberries, and raspberries are loaded with antioxidants.

- Leafy greens: Spinach, kale, and broccoli are rich in calcium and other bone-boosting nutrients.

Foods to Limit

1. **Salt** Excessive salt intake can lead to calcium loss through urine, weakening bones over time.

   Limiting processed and packaged foods, which are often high in sodium, can help reduce this risk.

Limit the following:

- Processed meats: Bacon, sausages, and deli meats.

- Packaged snacks: Chips, pretzels, and crackers.

- Canned soups and vegetables: Opt for low-sodium versions instead.

2. **Caffeine** High levels of caffeine can interfere with calcium absorption. While moderate coffee consumption is generally safe, excessive intake can be detrimental to bone health.

Limit the following:

- Coffee: Aim to limit coffee intake to no more than 2-3 cups per day.

- Energy drinks and sodas containing caffeine.

3. **Alcohol** Excessive alcohol consumption can interfere with the body's ability to absorb calcium and other nutrients. It also impairs the balance and coordination, increasing the risk of falls and fractures.

Limit the following:

- Alcoholic beverages: Particularly hard liquor and binge drinking.

Foods to Avoid

1. **Soft Drinks (Soda)** Sodas, particularly cola-type drinks, contain phosphoric acid, which can interfere with calcium absorption and lead to a loss of bone density. Additionally, sodas often replace healthier beverage options, such as milk or fortified plant-based drinks.

Avoid:

   o Cola drinks and other carbonated soft drinks

2. **High-Phosphorus Foods** While phosphorus is essential for bone health, too much phosphorus from processed foods can cause an imbalance, leading to calcium depletion. Avoid foods with added phosphates, such as processed meats and certain packaged foods.

Avoid:

   o Processed cheese, deli meats, and packaged baked goods with added phosphate preservatives

3. **Excessive Sugary Foods** A diet high in added sugars can lead to inflammation and reduce the intake of nutrient-dense foods essential for bone health. Excessive sugar can also contribute to obesity, which increases stress on bones and joints.

Avoid:

   o Candy, sugary desserts, and sweetened beverages (such as fruit juices with added sugar)

4. **Trans Fats** Trans fats, found in processed and fried foods, can promote inflammation and interfere with calcium absorption.

They also contribute to overall poor health, which can exacerbate osteoporosis symptoms.

Avoid:

- o Fried fast food, commercially baked goods (like cookies, cakes), and margarine with hydrogenated oils

Conclusion

For individuals with osteoporosis, focusing on a diet rich in calcium, vitamin D, protein, and anti-inflammatory nutrients is key to maintaining bone strength and reducing the risk of fractures. By limiting or avoiding foods that deplete calcium or cause inflammation—such as excessive salt, caffeine, alcohol, and sugary or processed foods—individuals can optimize their bone and joint health. A well-rounded, nutrient-dense diet can make a significant difference in managing osteoporosis and improving overall quality of life.

CHAPTER: 3

Supplements and Osteoporosis

While a balanced diet rich in calcium, vitamin D, and other nutrients is essential for maintaining bone health, many people, especially seniors, may not get enough of these key nutrients through food alone. This is where supplements play a crucial role. They help bridge the nutritional gaps and support bone health in individuals with osteoporosis or those at risk of developing it.

This comprehensive discussion will explore the various supplement options available, guidance on how to use them effectively for bone health, and the potential interactions and side effects that users should be aware of.

Understanding Supplement Options:

Several supplements are commonly recommended for the prevention and management of osteoporosis. The most important nutrients for bone health include calcium, vitamin D, magnesium, vitamin K, and other trace minerals. Each plays a unique role in maintaining bone strength and preventing bone loss. Below, we'll discuss these in detail.

1. Calcium

Supplement forms: Calcium supplements are available in two main forms: calcium carbonate and calcium citrate.

- **Calcium carbonate** contains a higher amount of elemental calcium and is often more affordable, but it requires stomach acid for absorption, meaning it should be taken with food.

- **Calcium citrate**, on the other hand, is absorbed more easily and can be taken with or without food, making it a better option for older adults or those with low stomach acid.

- **Recommended dosage:** The general recommendation for adults is around 1,000 mg of calcium per day, increasing to 1,200 mg for women over 50 and men over 70. It's important to note that calcium from supplements should be taken in divided doses, as the body can absorb only 500-600 mg at a time.

- **Natural food sources:** Dairy products, leafy greens, and fortified foods are good sources of calcium. However, for individuals who cannot get enough calcium from food, supplements are often necessary.

2. Vitamin D

- **Supplement forms:** Vitamin D supplements are available as **vitamin D2 (ergocalciferol)** and **vitamin D3 (cholecalciferol)**. Vitamin D3 is the preferred form, as it is more effective in raising and maintaining blood levels of vitamin D.

- **Recommended dosage:** The recommended daily intake for vitamin D varies depending on age, skin type, geographic location, and exposure to sunlight. For most adults, a daily intake of 600 to 800 IU is suggested, though individuals with low vitamin D levels may require higher doses. In many cases, a supplement of 1,000 to 2,000 IU per day is recommended to maintain optimal levels.

- **Natural sources:** While vitamin D is synthesized through sunlight exposure, it can also be found in fortified foods and fatty fish. However, many people—especially those living in areas with limited sunlight or those who spend most of their time indoors—may need supplements to reach adequate levels.

3. Magnesium

- **Supplement forms:** Magnesium supplements come in various forms, including **magnesium oxide, magnesium citrate, and magnesium glycinate**. Magnesium citrate and glycinate are better absorbed and tend to have fewer gastrointestinal side effects compared to magnesium oxide.

- **Recommended dosage:** The daily recommended intake for magnesium is around 320 mg for women and 420 mg for men. Supplements are often needed if dietary intake is insufficient.

- **Natural sources:** Foods rich in magnesium include leafy greens, nuts, seeds, whole grains, and legumes.

However, older adults, especially those with certain health conditions or on medications that reduce magnesium absorption, may require supplements.

4. Vitamin K

- **Supplement forms:** Vitamin K is available as **vitamin K1 (phylloquinone)** and **vitamin K2 (menaquinone)**. Vitamin K2 is thought to be more effective for bone health, as it activates osteocalcin, a protein involved in bone mineralization.

- **Recommended dosage:** The daily recommendation for vitamin K is 90 mcg for women and 120 mcg for men. However, higher doses of vitamin K2 may be beneficial for bone health, particularly for those with osteoporosis.

- **Natural sources:** Vitamin K1 is abundant in green leafy vegetables like spinach and kale, while K2 is found in fermented foods, such as natto (fermented soybeans), and in small amounts in animal products.

5. Other Trace Minerals (Zinc, Copper, and Boron)

Several trace minerals are also essential for maintaining bone health. **Zinc** is involved in bone tissue renewal, **copper** helps with collagen formation (which provides a framework for bone mineralization), and **boron** aids in the metabolism of calcium, magnesium, and vitamin D.

- **Recommended dosage:** While these minerals are needed in much smaller quantities than calcium or magnesium, they are still vital for bone health.

Zinc, for instance, has a recommended daily intake of 8 mg for women and 11 mg for men.

- **Natural sources:** These trace minerals can be found in a variety of foods, including nuts, seeds, seafood, and whole grains.

Guidance on Supplement Use for Bone Health

Supplements can be an effective tool in managing osteoporosis, but their use must be tailored to the individual's needs. Here are some key guidelines for using supplements effectively for bone health:

1. Consultation with Healthcare Providers

Before starting any supplements, it's crucial to consult with a healthcare provider.

A blood test can reveal deficiencies in calcium, vitamin D, or other key nutrients, and a doctor can recommend appropriate supplements and dosages. For individuals already taking medications, such as bisphosphonates for osteoporosis, supplements may need to be adjusted to avoid interactions.

2. Proper Timing and Dosage

- **Calcium:** As the body can absorb only 500-600 mg of calcium at a time, it is important to divide the total daily dose into two or more smaller doses.

  Calcium carbonate should be taken with meals, while calcium citrate can be taken at any time.

- **Vitamin D and Calcium Pairing:** It's essential to take vitamin D with calcium to maximize calcium absorption.

Many combination supplements are available that provide both nutrients in appropriate ratios.

3. Balanced Diet

While supplements can help fill nutritional gaps, they should not replace a healthy, balanced diet. Foods provide a variety of nutrients that work synergistically to promote bone health, so supplements should complement a nutrient-rich diet rather than act as a substitute.

4. Monitoring and Adjustments

Regular monitoring of bone density and blood levels of calcium and vitamin D is important for adjusting supplement doses as needed.

Too much calcium or vitamin D can lead to negative side effects, including kidney stones and hypercalcemia (excess calcium in the blood), so periodic testing is recommended.

Potential Interactions and Side Effects:

While supplements can provide critical support for bone health, it's important to be aware of potential interactions and side effects that can arise from improper use or over-supplementation.

1. Calcium Overload

Taking too much calcium from supplements, particularly in individuals who already consume a lot of calcium-rich foods, can lead to kidney stones or hypercalcemia.

This condition, marked by excessive calcium levels in the blood, can result in nausea, vomiting, confusion, and other serious health problems.

Risk factors:

- Overuse of calcium supplements in combination with calcium-rich foods.

- Taking high doses of calcium without regular monitoring.

2. Vitamin D Toxicity

While rare, vitamin D toxicity can occur if excessive amounts are taken over time. Symptoms of vitamin D toxicity include nausea, weakness, and an elevated risk of kidney damage due to excessive calcium absorption.

Risk factors:

- Taking very high doses of vitamin D supplements without regular monitoring of blood levels.

3. Medication Interactions

Supplements can interact with prescription medications, potentially reducing their efficacy or increasing side effects. For example:

- **Calcium supplements** can interfere with the absorption of thyroid medications, certain antibiotics, and bisphosphonates (commonly prescribed for osteoporosis).

- **Vitamin K supplements** may reduce the effectiveness of blood-thinning medications like warfarin. Individuals on these medications should consult their doctor before taking vitamin K supplements.

4. Gastrointestinal Side Effects

Some supplements, particularly calcium and magnesium, can cause gastrointestinal issues such as constipation or diarrhea, depending on the form and dosage.

Calcium carbonate is more likely to cause constipation, while magnesium supplements, especially in high doses, can have a laxative effect.

Solution: Choosing better-tolerated forms like calcium citrate and magnesium glycinate can help reduce these side effects.

Additionally, taking supplements with meals may lessen stomach discomfort.

5. Overlapping Supplements

Many multivitamins contain calcium, vitamin D, and magnesium, which can lead to over-supplementation if taken along with separate bone health supplements. It's important to read labels carefully and avoid taking overlapping products that exceed the recommended daily intake.

Conclusion

Supplements can be an important part of managing osteoporosis and promoting bone health, especially for individuals who may not get enough key nutrients from their diet. However, it's essential to approach supplementation with care, ensuring that dosages are appropriate and that potential interactions with medications or other supplements are considered. Consulting a healthcare provider, maintaining a balanced diet, and monitoring blood levels are crucial steps in safely and effectively using supplements to support strong bones and prevent fractures.

CALCIUM FORTIFIED BREAKFAST RECIPES:

Calcium-Rich Almond & Chia Pudding

Ingredients:

- 2 tablespoons chia seeds
- 1 cup unsweetened almond milk (calcium-fortified)
- 1 teaspoon vanilla extract
- 1/4 cup unsweetened almond yogurt
- 1 tablespoon sliced almonds
- 1/4 cup blueberries

Preparation:

1. In a bowl, combine chia seeds, almond milk, and vanilla extract. Stir well.

2. Let it sit in the fridge for at least 2-3 hours (or overnight).

3. Stir the mixture, then top with almond yogurt, sliced almonds, and blueberries before serving.

Number of servings: 1

Nutritional Information (per serving):

- Calories: 180
- Protein: 6g
- Fat: 12g
- Carbohydrates: 12g
- Calcium: 350mg
- Magnesium: 100mg
- Vitamin D: 100 IU
- Vitamin K: 8mcg

Cooking Time: 5 minutes prep + 3 hours chilling

Spinach and Mushroom Egg Scramble

Ingredients:

- 2 large eggs (vitamin D-fortified)
- 1/2 cup spinach (vitamin K-rich)
- 1/4 cup mushrooms (vitamin D-rich)
- 1 tablespoon olive oil
- 1 tablespoon low-fat feta cheese
- Salt and pepper to taste

Preparation:

1. Heat olive oil in a pan over medium heat.
2. Add mushrooms and spinach, sautéing until softened (about 3 minutes).
3. Beat the eggs in a bowl and pour them into the pan.
4. Stir continuously until eggs are scrambled and cooked through.
5. Top with feta cheese, season with salt and pepper, and serve.

Number of servings: 1

Nutritional Information (per serving):

- Calories: 210
- Protein: 14g
- Fat: 16g
- Carbohydrates: 3g
- Calcium: 150mg
- Magnesium: 60mg
- Vitamin D: 180 IU
- Vitamin K: 145mcg

Cooking Time: 10 minutes

Calcium-Fortified Oatmeal with Almond Butter

Ingredients:

- 1/2 cup oats
- 1 cup unsweetened almond milk (calcium-fortified)
- 1 tablespoon almond butter
- 1 tablespoon chia seeds
- 1/4 teaspoon cinnamon
- 1/4 cup raspberries

Preparation:

1. In a saucepan, bring almond milk to a gentle boil.

2. Stir in oats and cook for 5 minutes, stirring occasionally.

3. Once thickened, remove from heat and mix in almond butter, chia seeds, and cinnamon.

4. Top with raspberries before serving.

Number of servings: 1

Nutritional Information (per serving):

- Calories: 290
- Protein: 10g
- Fat: 12g
- Carbohydrates: 34g
- Calcium: 400mg
- Magnesium: 120mg
- Vitamin D: 100 IU
- Vitamin K: 5mcg

Cooking Time: 10 minutes

Kale and Avocado Smoothie

Ingredients:

- 1 cup kale leaves (vitamin K-rich)

- 1/2 avocado

- 1 cup unsweetened almond milk (calcium-fortified)

- 1 tablespoon chia seeds

- 1/2 banana

- 1 tablespoon almond butter

Preparation:

1. Combine all ingredients in a blender.

2. Blend until smooth and creamy.

3. Serve immediately.

Number of servings: 1

Nutritional Information (per serving):

- Calories: 320

- Protein: 7g

- Fat: 23g

- Carbohydrates: 22g

- Calcium: 350mg

- Magnesium: 140mg

- Vitamin D: 100 IU

- Vitamin K: 200mcg

Cooking Time: 5 minutes

Greek Yogurt Parfait with Nuts and Berries

Ingredients:

- 1/2 cup Greek yogurt (calcium-rich)

- 1 tablespoon chia seeds

- 1/4 cup mixed berries (blueberries, raspberries)

- 1 tablespoon walnuts (magnesium-rich)

- 1 tablespoon unsweetened almond butter

Preparation:

1. Layer Greek yogurt at the bottom of a bowl or glass.

2. Add chia seeds, berries, walnuts, and almond butter on top.

3. Serve immediately.

Number of servings: 1

Nutritional Information (per serving):

- Calories: 250

- Protein: 12g

- Fat: 14g

- Carbohydrates: 20g

- Calcium: 300mg

- Magnesium: 110mg

- Vitamin D: 40 IU

- Vitamin K: 10mcg

Cooking Time: 5 minutes

Cottage Cheese with Flaxseeds and Strawberries

Ingredients:

- 1/2 cup low-fat cottage cheese (calcium-rich)
- 1 tablespoon flaxseeds (magnesium-rich)
- 1/4 cup sliced strawberries
- 1 tablespoon chopped almonds

Preparation:

1. In a bowl, add cottage cheese.
2. Sprinkle flaxseeds, almonds, and top with sliced strawberries.
3. Serve chilled.

Number of servings: 1

Nutritional Information (per serving):

- Calories: 180
- Protein: 14g
- Fat: 8g
- Carbohydrates: 10g
- Calcium: 250mg
- Magnesium: 80mg
- Vitamin D: 30 IU
- Vitamin K: 6mcg

Cooking Time: 5 minutes

Scrambled Tofu with Spinach and Sunflower Seeds

Ingredients:

- 1/2 cup firm tofu (calcium-fortified)

- 1/2 cup spinach (vitamin K-rich)

- 1 tablespoon sunflower seeds

- 1 teaspoon olive oil

- Salt and pepper to taste

Preparation:

1. Crumble tofu and set aside.

2. Heat olive oil in a pan over medium heat, add spinach, and cook until wilted.

3. Add tofu to the pan and cook for 5 minutes, stirring frequently.

4. Season with salt and pepper, sprinkle sunflower seeds on top, and serve.

Number of servings: 1

Nutritional Information (per serving):

- Calories: 210

- Protein: 12g

- Fat: 14g

- Carbohydrates: 6g

- Calcium: 180mg

- Magnesium: 85mg

- Vitamin D: 50 IU

- Vitamin K: 100mcg

Cooking Time: 10 minutes

Chia and Flaxseed Breakfast Muffins

Ingredients:

- 1/2 cup almond flour
- 2 tablespoons chia seeds
- 2 tablespoons flaxseeds (ground)
- 1 egg (vitamin D-rich)
- 1/4 cup unsweetened almond milk (calcium-fortified)
- 1/2 teaspoon baking powder
- 1/4 teaspoon cinnamon

Preparation:

1. Preheat the oven to 350°F (175°C).
2. In a bowl, combine almond flour, chia seeds, flaxseeds, baking powder, and cinnamon.
3. In a separate bowl, whisk together the egg and almond milk.
4. Combine the wet and dry ingredients, mixing until smooth.
5. Pour into muffin tins and bake for 15 minutes.

Number of servings: 4 (1 muffin per serving)

Nutritional Information (per serving):

- Calories: 120
- Protein: 6g
- Fat: 9g
- Carbohydrates: 5g
- Calcium: 100mg
- Magnesium: 50mg
- Vitamin D: 40 IU
- Vitamin K: 2mcg

Cooking Time: 20 minutes

Avocado and Sardine Toast

Ingredients:

- 1 slice whole grain bread
- 1/2 avocado
- 1 small can of sardines in water (drained)
- 1 teaspoon lemon juice
- Pinch of salt and pepper

Preparation:

1. Toast the whole grain bread.
2. Mash avocado in a bowl and mix in lemon juice, salt, and pepper.
3. Spread avocado mash on the toast and top with sardines.
4. Serve immediately.

Number of servings: 1

Nutritional Information (per serving):

- Calories: 300
- Protein: 16g
- Fat: 22g
- Carbohydrates: 18g
- Calcium: 200mg
- Magnesium: 70mg
- Vitamin D: 100 IU
- Vitamin K: 15mcg

Cooking Time: 5 minutes

Baked Eggs with Spinach and Mushrooms

Ingredients:

- 2 large eggs (vitamin D-rich)
- 1/2 cup spinach (vitamin K-rich)
- 1/4 cup mushrooms
- 1 tablespoon olive oil
- Salt and pepper to taste

Preparation:

1. Preheat the oven to 350°F (175°C).
2. Sauté spinach and mushrooms in olive oil until softened.
3. Divide spinach-mushroom mixture into two ramekins, then crack an egg on top of each.
4. Bake for 10-12 minutes until the eggs are set.
5. Season with salt and pepper, and serve.

Number of servings: 1

Nutritional Information (per serving):

- Calories: 220
- Protein: 14g
- Fat: 16g
- Carbohydrates: 4g
- Calcium: 120mg
- Magnesium: 50mg
- Vitamin D: 160 IU
- Vitamin K: 180mcg

Cooking Time: 15 minutes

Buckwheat Pancakes with Blueberries

Ingredients:

- 1/2 cup buckwheat flour
- 1 egg
- 1/4 cup unsweetened almond milk (calcium-fortified)
- 1/4 teaspoon baking powder
- 1/4 cup blueberries
- 1 teaspoon olive oil

Preparation:

1. In a bowl, whisk together buckwheat flour, baking powder, egg, and almond milk until smooth.
2. Heat a non-stick pan with olive oil over medium heat.
3. Pour 1/4 cup of batter into the pan and cook until bubbles form on the surface, then flip and cook the other side.
4. Top with fresh blueberries and serve.

Number of servings: 2

Nutritional Information (per serving):

- Calories: 180
- Protein: 6g
- Fat: 5g
- Carbohydrates: 30g
- Calcium: 120mg
- Magnesium: 40mg
- Vitamin D: 40 IU
- Vitamin K: 5mcg

Cooking Time: 15 minutes

Sunflower Seed and Spinach Smoothie

Ingredients:

- 1 cup spinach (vitamin K-rich)
- 1 tablespoon sunflower seeds (magnesium-rich)
- 1/2 avocado
- 1/2 cup unsweetened almond milk (calcium-fortified)
- 1/4 cup strawberries

Preparation:

1. Add all ingredients into a blender.
2. Blend until smooth and creamy.
3. Serve immediately.

Number of servings: 1

Nutritional Information (per serving):

- Calories: 260
- Protein: 5g
- Fat: 21g
- Carbohydrates: 15g
- Calcium: 180mg
- Magnesium: 80mg
- Vitamin D: 40 IU
- Vitamin K: 250mcg

Cooking Time: 5 minutes

Quinoa Breakfast Bowl with Almonds and Berries

Ingredients:

- 1/2 cup cooked quinoa
- 1 tablespoon chia seeds
- 1 tablespoon sliced almonds
- 1/4 cup mixed berries (blueberries, strawberries)
- 1/4 cup unsweetened almond milk (calcium-fortified)

Preparation:

1. In a bowl, combine cooked quinoa, chia seeds, and almond milk.
2. Top with sliced almonds and mixed berries.
3. Serve immediately.

Number of servings: 1

Nutritional Information (per serving):

- Calories: 250
- Protein: 8g
- Fat: 10g
- Carbohydrates: 30g
- Calcium: 150mg
- Magnesium: 90mg
- Vitamin D: 40 IU
- Vitamin K: 10mcg

Cooking Time: 10 minutes

Sweet Potato and Kale Hash

Ingredients:

- 1 small sweet potato, diced
- 1 cup kale (vitamin K-rich)
- 1 tablespoon olive oil
- 1/4 teaspoon cumin
- Salt and pepper to taste

Preparation:

1. Heat olive oil in a pan over medium heat.
2. Add diced sweet potato and sauté until tender (about 10 minutes).
3. Add kale and cumin, cooking until kale is wilted.
4. Season with salt and pepper, and serve.

Number of servings: 1

Nutritional Information (per serving):

- Calories: 180
- Protein: 4g
- Fat: 8g
- Carbohydrates: 25g
- Calcium: 120mg
- Magnesium: 40mg
- Vitamin D: 0 IU
- Vitamin K: 300mcg

Cooking Time: 15 minutes

Apple-Cinnamon Chia Pudding

Ingredients:

- 1/4 cup chia seeds
- 1 cup unsweetened almond milk (calcium-fortified)
- 1/2 apple, diced
- 1/2 teaspoon cinnamon

Preparation:

1. In a bowl, mix chia seeds, almond milk, and cinnamon.
2. Refrigerate for at least 2-3 hours (or overnight).
3. Top with diced apple before serving.

Number of servings: 1

Nutritional Information (per serving):

- Calories: 200
- Protein: 5g
- Fat: 11g
- Carbohydrates: 22g
- Calcium: 300mg
- Magnesium: 90mg
- Vitamin D: 100 IU
- Vitamin K: 3mcg

Cooking Time: 5 minutes prep + 3 hours chilling

These recipes provide nutrient-dense, delicious breakfast options that are easy to prepare and designed to support bone health for seniors with osteoporosis while also being diabetes- and heart-friendly.

LUNCH RECIPES FOR STRONG BONES:

Grilled Salmon and Kale Salad

Ingredients:

- 1 salmon fillet (4 oz)

- 2 cups kale (vitamin K-rich)

- 1 tablespoon olive oil

- 1 tablespoon lemon juice

- 1 tablespoon sunflower seeds (magnesium-rich)

- Salt and pepper to taste

Preparation:

1. Preheat grill or pan to medium heat.

2. Season the salmon with salt and pepper. Grill for 4-5 minutes on each side until fully cooked.

3. Toss the kale with olive oil, lemon juice, and sunflower seeds.

4. Top the kale salad with grilled salmon and serve.

Number of servings: 1

Nutritional Information (per serving):

- Calories: 380

- Protein: 28g

- Fat: 24g

- Carbohydrates: 6g

- Calcium: 150mg

- Magnesium: 100mg

- Vitamin D: 400 IU

- Vitamin K: 250mcg

Cooking Time: 15 minutes

Quinoa and Spinach Stuffed Bell Peppers

Ingredients:

- 2 bell peppers, halved and seeded

- 1/2 cup cooked quinoa

- 1/2 cup spinach (vitamin K-rich)

- 1/4 cup feta cheese (calcium-rich)

- 1 tablespoon olive oil

- Salt and pepper to taste

Preparation:

1. Preheat oven to 375°F (190°C).

2. Sauté spinach in olive oil until wilted. Mix in quinoa and feta cheese.

3. Stuff the mixture into the bell pepper halves and place them in a baking dish.

4. Bake for 20 minutes until peppers are tender.

Number of servings: 2

Nutritional Information (per serving):

- Calories: 280

- Protein: 8g

- Fat: 14g

- Carbohydrates: 25g

- Calcium: 200mg

- Magnesium: 70mg

- Vitamin D: 40 IU

- Vitamin K: 220mcg

Cooking Time: 30 minutes

Lentil and Kale Soup

Ingredients:

- 1/2 cup dry lentils
- 1 cup kale (vitamin K-rich)
- 1/2 onion, diced
- 1 garlic clove, minced
- 1 tablespoon olive oil
- 4 cups low-sodium vegetable broth
- 1 teaspoon cumin
- Salt and pepper to taste

Preparation:

1. Heat olive oil in a pot over medium heat. Add onion and garlic, sautéing until softened.
2. Add lentils, vegetable broth, cumin, salt, and pepper. Bring to a boil, then reduce heat and simmer for 20 minutes.
3. Stir in kale and cook for an additional 5 minutes. Serve hot.

Number of servings: 2

Nutritional Information (per serving):

- Calories: 250
- Protein: 13g
- Fat: 8g
- Carbohydrates: 34g
- Calcium: 150mg
- Magnesium: 75mg
- Vitamin D: 0 IU
- Vitamin K: 350mcg

Cooking Time: 30 minutes

Baked Cod with Broccoli and Almonds

Ingredients:

- 1 cod fillet (4 oz)

- 1 cup broccoli florets (vitamin K-rich)

- 1 tablespoon sliced almonds (magnesium-rich)

- 1 tablespoon olive oil

- 1 tablespoon lemon juice

- Salt and pepper to taste

Preparation:

1. Preheat oven to 375°F (190°C).

2. Place cod on a baking sheet, drizzle with olive oil and lemon juice, and season with salt and pepper. Bake for 12-15 minutes until cooked through.

3. Steam the broccoli until tender, then top with sliced almonds.

4. Serve the cod alongside the broccoli.

Number of servings: 1

Nutritional Information (per serving):

- Calories: 320

- Protein: 25g

- Fat: 18g

- Carbohydrates: 10g

- Calcium: 180mg

- Magnesium: 80mg

- Vitamin D: 200 IU

- Vitamin K: 180mcg

Cooking Time: 20 minutes

Turkey Lettuce Wraps with Avocado

Ingredients:

- 4 large romaine lettuce leaves
- 4 oz ground turkey (lean)
- 1/2 avocado, sliced
- 1/4 cup shredded carrots
- 1 tablespoon olive oil
- 1 teaspoon soy sauce (low-sodium)
- Salt and pepper to taste

Preparation:

1. Heat olive oil in a skillet over medium heat. Add ground turkey, cooking until browned and fully cooked.

2. Stir in soy sauce, salt, and pepper.

3. Place cooked turkey into lettuce leaves, top with avocado slices and shredded carrots. Wrap and serve.

Number of servings: 2

Nutritional Information (per serving):

- Calories: 250
- Protein: 19g
- Fat: 17g
- Carbohydrates: 7g
- Calcium: 50mg
- Magnesium: 50mg
- Vitamin D: 0 IU
- Vitamin K: 100mcg

Cooking Time: 15 minutes

Grilled Chicken and Spinach Salad with Walnuts

Ingredients:

- 1 grilled chicken breast (4 oz)

- 2 cups baby spinach (vitamin K-rich)

- 1 tablespoon chopped walnuts (magnesium-rich)

- 1 tablespoon olive oil

- 1 tablespoon balsamic vinegar

- 1/4 cup cherry tomatoes

- Salt and pepper to taste

Preparation:

1. Grill the chicken breast until fully cooked, about 6-8 minutes per side.

2. In a large bowl, toss spinach, cherry tomatoes, walnuts, olive oil, and balsamic vinegar.

3. Slice the grilled chicken and add to the salad. Season with salt and pepper, then serve.

Number of servings: 1

Nutritional Information (per serving):

- Calories: 340

- Protein: 34g

- Fat: 22g

- Carbohydrates: 6g

- Calcium: 120mg

- Magnesium: 90mg

- Vitamin D: 0 IU

- Vitamin K: 300mcg

Cooking Time: 20 minutes

Quinoa and Chickpea Bowl with Tahini Dressing

Ingredients:

- 1/2 cup cooked quinoa
- 1/2 cup canned chickpeas (rinsed)
- 1/4 cup cucumber, diced
- 1/4 cup cherry tomatoes, halved
- 1 tablespoon tahini
- 1 tablespoon lemon juice
- 1 tablespoon olive oil
- Salt and pepper to taste

Preparation:

1. In a bowl, combine cooked quinoa, chickpeas, cucumber, and tomatoes.

2. Whisk together tahini, lemon juice, olive oil, salt, and pepper to make the dressing.

3. Drizzle the dressing over the quinoa mixture and toss well before serving.

Number of servings: 2

Nutritional Information (per serving):

- Calories: 320
- Protein: 12g
- Fat: 14g
- Carbohydrates: 38g
- Calcium: 100mg
- Magnesium: 85mg
- Vitamin D: 0 IU
- Vitamin K: 10mcg

Cooking Time: 15 minutes

Tofu Stir-Fry with Broccoli and Mushrooms

Ingredients:

- 1/2 cup firm tofu (calcium-rich)

- 1 cup broccoli florets (vitamin K-rich)

- 1/2 cup sliced mushrooms (vitamin D-rich)

- 1 tablespoon soy sauce (low-sodium)

- 1 tablespoon olive oil

- 1 garlic clove, minced

- Salt and pepper to taste

Preparation:

1. Heat olive oil in a skillet over medium heat. Add tofu and cook until golden on all sides, about 5-7 minutes.

2. Add garlic, broccoli, mushrooms, and soy sauce, sautéing until vegetables are tender, about 5 minutes.

3. Season with salt and pepper, and serve hot.

Number of servings: 1

Nutritional Information (per serving):

- Calories: 260

- Protein: 14g

- Fat: 16g

- Carbohydrates: 16g

- Calcium: 200mg

- Magnesium: 85mg

- Vitamin D: 150 IU

- Vitamin K: 180mcg

Cooking Time: 15 minutes

Grilled Shrimp with Spinach and Avocado Salad

Ingredients:

- 6 large shrimp (peeled and deveined)
- 2 cups spinach (vitamin K-rich)
- 1/2 avocado, sliced
- 1 tablespoon olive oil
- 1 tablespoon lemon juice
- Salt and pepper to taste

Preparation:

1. Grill shrimp for 2-3 minutes on each side, until opaque.
2. In a bowl, toss spinach, avocado slices, olive oil, lemon juice, salt, and pepper.
3. Top the salad with grilled shrimp and serve.

Number of servings: 1

Nutritional Information (per serving):

- Calories: 320
- Protein: 20g
- Fat: 22g
- Carbohydrates: 8g
- Calcium: 120mg
- Magnesium: 70mg
- Vitamin D: 50 IU
- Vitamin K: 280mcg

Cooking Time: 10 minutes

Cauliflower and Chickpea Curry

Ingredients:

- 1 cup cauliflower florets
- 1/2 cup canned chickpeas (rinsed)
- 1/4 cup diced tomatoes
- 1/2 onion, diced
- 1 garlic clove, minced
- 1 tablespoon curry powder
- 1 tablespoon olive oil
- 1/2 cup low-sodium vegetable broth
- Salt and pepper to taste

Preparation:

1. Heat olive oil in a pot over medium heat. Add onion and garlic, sautéing until softened.

2. Stir in curry powder, chickpeas, cauliflower, diced tomatoes, and vegetable broth. Bring to a boil, then reduce heat and simmer for 15 minutes.

3. Season with salt and pepper, and serve.

Number of servings: 2

Nutritional Information (per serving):

- Calories: 230
- Protein: 8g
- Fat: 10g
- Carbohydrates: 26g
- Calcium: 70mg
- Magnesium: 60mg
- Vitamin D: 0 IU
- Vitamin K: 40mcg

Cooking Time: 20 minutes

Eggplant and Tomato Stew

Ingredients:

- 1 small eggplant, diced
- 1/2 cup diced tomatoes
- 1 garlic clove, minced
- 1 tablespoon olive oil
- 1/4 teaspoon cumin
- Salt and pepper to taste

Preparation:

1. Heat olive oil in a pot over medium heat. Add garlic and cumin, sautéing for 1 minute.
2. Add diced eggplant and tomatoes, cooking until eggplant softens, about 10 minutes.
3. Season with salt and pepper, and serve hot.

Number of servings: 1

Nutritional Information (per serving):

- Calories: 180
- Protein: 3g
- Fat: 11g
- Carbohydrates: 20g
- Calcium: 60mg
- Magnesium: 45mg
- Vitamin D: 0 IU
- Vitamin K: 20mcg

Cooking Time: 15 minutes

Zucchini Noodles with Pesto

Ingredients:

- 1 large zucchini, spiralized

- 1 tablespoon pesto sauce (homemade or store-bought, low sodium)

- 1 tablespoon olive oil

- 1 tablespoon grated Parmesan cheese (calcium-rich)

Preparation:

1. Heat olive oil in a skillet over medium heat.

2. Add zucchini noodles and cook for 2-3 minutes until slightly tender.

3. Toss with pesto sauce and sprinkle with Parmesan cheese before serving.

Number of servings: 1

Nutritional Information (per serving):

- Calories: 210

- Protein: 6g

- Fat: 18g

- Carbohydrates: 7g

- Calcium: 100mg

- Magnesium: 40mg

- Vitamin D: 0 IU

- Vitamin K: 25mcg

Cooking Time: 10 minutes

Spinach and Feta Stuffed Portobello Mushrooms

Ingredients:

- 2 large Portobello mushrooms

- 1/2 cup spinach (vitamin K-rich)

- 1/4 cup feta cheese (calcium-rich)

- 1 tablespoon olive oil

- Salt and pepper to taste

Preparation:

1. Preheat oven to 375°F (190°C).

2. Remove stems from mushrooms and brush with olive oil.

3. Sauté spinach in olive oil until wilted, then mix with feta cheese.

4. Stuff the mushroom caps with the spinach and feta mixture.

5. Bake for 15 minutes, until mushrooms are tender.

Number of servings: 2

Nutritional Information (per serving):

- Calories: 200

- Protein: 8g

- Fat: 16g

- Carbohydrates: 6g

- Calcium: 150mg

- Magnesium: 45mg

- Vitamin D: 30 IU

- Vitamin K: 200mcg

Cooking Time: 20 minutes

Grilled Asparagus with Tofu and Tahini Sauce

Ingredients:

- 6 asparagus spears
- 1/2 cup firm tofu (calcium-rich)
- 1 tablespoon tahini
- 1 tablespoon lemon juice
- 1 tablespoon olive oil
- Salt and pepper to taste

Preparation:

1. Grill or roast the asparagus for 5-7 minutes until tender.
2. Sear the tofu in a hot pan with olive oil until golden on both sides.
3. Whisk together tahini, lemon juice, salt, and pepper to create the sauce.
4. Serve tofu and asparagus drizzled with tahini sauce.

Number of servings: 1

Nutritional Information (per serving):

- Calories: 280
- Protein: 12g
- Fat: 22g
- Carbohydrates: 10g
- Calcium: 220mg
- Magnesium: 80mg
- Vitamin D: 0 IU
- Vitamin K: 100mcg

Cooking Time: 15 minutes

These recipes are easy to prepare, nutrient-dense, and focused on enhancing bone health, while being both heart- and diabetes-friendly for seniors managing osteoporosis.

Dinner recipes:

Lemon Garlic Baked Chicken with Roasted Brussels Sprouts

Ingredients:

- 1 chicken breast (4 oz)
- 1 cup Brussels sprouts, halved (vitamin K-rich)
- 1 tablespoon olive oil
- 1 tablespoon lemon juice
- 2 garlic cloves, minced
- Salt and pepper to taste

Preparation:

1. Preheat oven to 375°F (190°C).

2. Toss Brussels sprouts with olive oil, salt, and pepper. Place them on a baking sheet.

3. Rub chicken breast with garlic and lemon juice, season with salt and pepper. Place on the same baking sheet.

4. Bake for 25-30 minutes, until the chicken is fully cooked and the Brussels sprouts are golden brown.

Number of servings: 1

Nutritional Information (per serving):

- Calories: 320
- Protein: 35g
- Fat: 14g
- Carbohydrates: 10g
- Calcium: 60mg
- Magnesium: 50mg
- Vitamin D: 0 IU
- Vitamin K: 220mcg

Cooking Time: 30 minutes

Grilled Mackerel with Steamed Spinach

Ingredients:

- 1 mackerel fillet (4 oz, vitamin D-rich)
- 2 cups spinach (vitamin K-rich)
- 1 tablespoon olive oil
- 1 tablespoon lemon juice
- 1 garlic clove, minced
- Salt and pepper to taste

Preparation:

1. Preheat the grill or pan over medium heat.
2. Rub the mackerel fillet with olive oil, garlic, lemon juice, salt, and pepper.
3. Grill the mackerel for 4-5 minutes per side until cooked through.
4. Steam spinach for 3-4 minutes until wilted. Serve together.

Number of servings: 1

Nutritional Information (per serving):

- Calories: 360
- Protein: 25g
- Fat: 24g
- Carbohydrates: 6g
- Calcium: 150mg
- Magnesium: 75mg
- Vitamin D: 450 IU
- Vitamin K: 300mcg

Cooking Time: 15 minutes

Zucchini Noodles with Garlic Shrimp

Ingredients:

- 1 zucchini, spiralized
- 6 large shrimp (peeled and deveined)
- 1 tablespoon olive oil
- 2 garlic cloves, minced
- 1 tablespoon lemon juice
- 1 tablespoon chopped parsley
- Salt and pepper to taste

Preparation:

1. Heat olive oil in a skillet over medium heat. Add garlic and cook for 1 minute.

2. Add shrimp and cook for 2-3 minutes per side until pink and opaque.

3. Toss zucchini noodles in with the shrimp and cook for 2-3 minutes until tender.

4. Season with lemon juice, parsley, salt, and pepper.

Number of servings: 1

Nutritional Information (per serving):

- Calories: 250
- Protein: 25g
- Fat: 14g
- Carbohydrates: 8g
- Calcium: 100mg
- Magnesium: 60mg
- Vitamin D: 20 IU
- Vitamin K: 50mcg

Cooking Time: 10 minutes

Baked Halibut with Almond-Crusted Asparagus

Ingredients:

- 1 halibut fillet (4 oz, vitamin D-rich)
- 6 asparagus spears (vitamin K-rich)
- 1 tablespoon almond flour
- 1 tablespoon olive oil
- 1 teaspoon lemon zest
- Salt and pepper to taste

Preparation:

1. Preheat oven to 375°F (190°C).

2. Place halibut fillet on a baking sheet, drizzle with olive oil, lemon zest, and season with salt and pepper.

3. Toss the asparagus spears with olive oil, almond flour, and a pinch of salt. Place them on the same baking sheet as the halibut.

4. Bake for 12-15 minutes until the halibut is cooked through and the asparagus is tender and lightly golden.

5. Serve together with a drizzle of lemon juice.

Number of servings: 1

Nutritional Information (per serving):

- Calories: 320
- Protein: 28g
- Fat: 18g
- Carbohydrates: 6g
- Calcium: 120mg
- Magnesium: 70mg
- Vitamin D: 400 IU
- Vitamin K: 130mcg

Cooking Time: 15 minutes

Turkey and Kale Stir-Fry

Ingredients:

- 4 oz ground turkey (lean)
- 2 cups kale, chopped (vitamin K-rich)
- 1/2 onion, diced
- 1 tablespoon olive oil
- 1 tablespoon low-sodium soy sauce
- 1 garlic clove, minced
- Salt and pepper to taste

Preparation:

1. Heat olive oil in a skillet over medium heat. Add onion and garlic, sauté until softened.

2. Add ground turkey and cook until browned, about 6-8 minutes.

3. Stir in chopped kale and soy sauce, cooking for an additional 3-4 minutes until the kale is wilted.

4. Season with salt and pepper and serve hot.

Number of servings: 1

Nutritional Information (per serving):

- Calories: 280
- Protein: 30g
- Fat: 14g
- Carbohydrates: 6g
- Calcium: 100mg
- Magnesium: 60mg
- Vitamin D: 0 IU
- Vitamin K: 250mcg

Cooking Time: 15 minutes

Baked Tofu with Broccoli and Sesame Seeds

Ingredients:

- 1/2 cup firm tofu (calcium-fortified)

- 1 cup broccoli florets (vitamin K-rich)

- 1 tablespoon olive oil

- 1 tablespoon sesame seeds (magnesium-rich)

- 1 tablespoon soy sauce (low-sodium)

- 1 teaspoon sesame oil

- Salt and pepper to taste

Preparation:

1. Preheat oven to 375°F (190°C).

2. Toss broccoli florets with olive oil, salt, and pepper. Place on a baking sheet.

3. Cut tofu into cubes and toss with soy sauce and sesame oil. Add to the baking sheet.

4. Bake for 15-20 minutes until the tofu is golden and the broccoli is tender.

5. Sprinkle sesame seeds on top before serving.

Number of servings: 1

Nutritional Information (per serving):

- Calories: 300

- Protein: 12g

- Fat: 20g

- Carbohydrates: 12g

- Calcium: 180mg

- Magnesium: 90mg

- Vitamin D: 0 IU

- Vitamin K: 220mcg

Cooking Time: 20 minutes

Garlic and Lemon Roasted Cauliflower with Grilled Chicken

Ingredients:

- 1/2 head cauliflower, cut into florets

- 1 chicken breast (4 oz)

- 1 tablespoon olive oil

- 1 garlic clove, minced

- 1 tablespoon lemon juice

- Salt and pepper to taste

Preparation:

1. Preheat oven to 400°F (200°C).

2. Toss cauliflower florets with olive oil, garlic, lemon juice, salt, and pepper. Spread on a baking sheet and roast for 20-25 minutes until golden and tender.

3. Grill the chicken breast for 6-8 minutes per side until fully cooked.

4. Serve the roasted cauliflower alongside the grilled chicken.

Number of servings: 1

Nutritional Information (per serving):

- Calories: 350

- Protein: 35g

- Fat: 18g

- Carbohydrates: 10g

- Calcium: 50mg

- Magnesium: 55mg

- Vitamin D: 0 IU

- Vitamin K: 30mcg

Cooking Time: 30 minutes

Spinach and Feta-Stuffed Chicken Breast

Ingredients:

- 1 chicken breast (4 oz)
- 1/2 cup spinach (vitamin K-rich)
- 2 tablespoons feta cheese (calcium-rich)
- 1 tablespoon olive oil
- 1 garlic clove, minced
- Salt and pepper to taste

Preparation:

1. Preheat oven to 375°F (190°C).
2. In a skillet, sauté spinach and garlic in olive oil until wilted. Remove from heat and mix with feta cheese.
3. Cut a pocket into the side of the chicken breast and stuff with the spinach-feta mixture.
4. Place chicken in a baking dish and bake for 20-25 minutes until cooked through.

Number of servings: 1

Nutritional Information (per serving):

- Calories: 350
- Protein: 37g
- Fat: 18g
- Carbohydrates: 3g
- Calcium: 200mg
- Magnesium: 50mg
- Vitamin D: 30 IU
- Vitamin K: 200mcg

Cooking Time: 30 minutes

Sautéed Salmon with Wilted Spinach and Garlic

Ingredients:

- 1 salmon fillet (4 oz, vitamin D-rich)

- 2 cups spinach (vitamin K-rich)

- 1 tablespoon olive oil

- 2 garlic cloves, minced

- 1 tablespoon lemon juice

- Salt and pepper to taste

Preparation:

1. Heat half of the olive oil in a pan over medium heat. Season the salmon with salt and pepper, then cook for 4-5 minutes per side until fully cooked.

2. In a separate pan, heat the remaining olive oil and garlic. Add spinach and cook until wilted, about 3 minutes.

3. Serve the salmon with the wilted spinach and a drizzle of lemon juice.

Number of servings: 1

Nutritional Information (per serving):

- Calories: 350

- Protein: 25g

- Fat: 26g

- Carbohydrates: 4g

- Calcium: 120mg

- Magnesium: 60mg

- Vitamin D: 450 IU

- Vitamin K: 300mcg

Cooking Time: 15 minutes

Roasted Eggplant and Chickpea Salad

Ingredients:

- 1 small eggplant, diced
- 1/2 cup cooked chickpeas (magnesium-rich)
- 1 tablespoon olive oil
- 1 tablespoon lemon juice
- 1 tablespoon chopped parsley
- Salt and pepper to taste

Preparation:

1. Preheat oven to 400°F (200°C).
2. Toss eggplant with olive oil, salt, and pepper. Roast on a baking sheet for 20-25 minutes until tender.
3. Mix roasted eggplant with cooked chickpeas, lemon juice, and parsley. Serve warm.

Number of servings: 1

Nutritional Information (per serving):

- Calories: 250
- Protein: 6g
- Fat: 14g
- Carbohydrates: 30g
- Calcium: 60mg
- Magnesium: 80mg
- Vitamin D: 0 IU
- Vitamin K: 20mcg

Cooking Time: 30 minutes

Shrimp and Avocado Salad

Ingredients:

- 6 large shrimp (peeled and deveined)

- 1/2 avocado, diced

- 1 cup mixed greens (vitamin K-rich)

- 1 tablespoon olive oil

- 1 tablespoon lemon juice

- Salt and pepper to taste

Preparation:

1. Grill or sauté shrimp for 2-3 minutes per side until pink and opaque.

2. In a bowl, combine mixed greens, avocado, olive oil, and lemon juice.

3. Top the salad with cooked shrimp and season with salt and pepper.

Number of servings: 1

Nutritional Information (per serving):

- Calories: 320

- Protein: 20g

- Fat: 24g

- Carbohydrates: 8g

- Calcium: 100mg

- Magnesium: 60mg

- Vitamin D: 20 IU

- Vitamin K: 150mcg

Cooking Time: 10 minutes

Cabbage and Mushroom Stir-Fry with Tofu

Ingredients:

- 1/2 cup firm tofu (calcium-fortified)
- 1 cup cabbage, shredded
- 1/2 cup sliced mushrooms (vitamin D-rich)
- 1 tablespoon olive oil
- 1 tablespoon soy sauce (low-sodium)
- Salt and pepper to taste

Preparation:

1. Heat olive oil in a pan over medium heat. Add tofu and cook until golden on all sides.
2. Add mushrooms and cabbage to the pan and cook until softened, about 5 minutes.
3. Stir in soy sauce and season with salt and pepper. Serve warm.

Number of servings: 1

Nutritional Information (per serving):

- Calories: 280
- Protein: 12g
- Fat: 18g
- Carbohydrates: 14g
- Calcium: 180mg
- Magnesium: 75mg
- Vitamin D: 150 IU
- Vitamin K: 90mcg

Cooking Time: 15 minutes

Baked Sweet Potatoes with Tahini Drizzle

Ingredients:

- 1 small sweet potato, halved
- 1 tablespoon tahini
- 1 tablespoon lemon juice
- 1 teaspoon olive oil
- Salt and pepper to taste

Preparation:

1. Preheat oven to 400°F (200°C).

2. Place sweet potato halves on a baking sheet and drizzle with olive oil. Bake for 25-30 minutes until tender.

3. Mix tahini, lemon juice, salt, and pepper. Drizzle over the baked sweet potatoes before serving.

Number of servings: 1

Nutritional Information (per serving):

- Calories: 250
- Protein: 4g
- Fat: 12g
- Carbohydrates: 34g
- Calcium: 60mg
- Magnesium: 70mg
- Vitamin D: 0 IU
- Vitamin K: 15mcg

Cooking Time: 30 minutes

Grilled Veggie Skewers with Chicken

Ingredients:

- 1 chicken breast (4 oz)
- 1/2 zucchini, sliced
- 1/2 red bell pepper, chopped
- 1/2 onion, chopped
- 1 tablespoon olive oil
- 1 tablespoon lemon juice
- Salt and pepper to taste

Preparation:

1. Preheat grill or broiler.
2. Thread chicken and vegetables onto skewers.
3. Drizzle with olive oil and lemon juice, season with salt and pepper.
4. Grill for 10-12 minutes, turning occasionally, until chicken is cooked through.

Number of servings: 1

Nutritional Information (per serving):

- Calories: 320
- Protein: 34g
- Fat: 16g
- Carbohydrates: 10g
- Calcium: 50mg
- Magnesium: 60mg
- Vitamin D: 0 IU
- Vitamin K: 20mcg

Cooking Time: 15 minutes

Baked Cod with Lemon and Spinach

Ingredients:

- 1 cod fillet (4 oz)
- 2 cups spinach (vitamin K-rich)
- 1 tablespoon olive oil
- 1 tablespoon lemon juice
- 1 garlic clove, minced
- Salt and pepper to taste

Preparation:

1. Preheat oven to 375°F (190°C).
2. Place cod on a baking sheet, drizzle with olive oil, lemon juice, garlic, salt, and pepper.
3. Bake for 12-15 minutes until cod is cooked through.
4. Steam spinach and serve alongside the cod.

Number of servings: 1

Nutritional Information (per serving):

- Calories: 280
- Protein: 25g
- Fat: 16g
- Carbohydrates: 6g
- Calcium: 120mg
- Magnesium: 60mg
- Vitamin D: 200 IU
- Vitamin K: 200mcg

Cooking Time: 20 minutes

These dinner recipes are packed with essential nutrients to support bone health, while being diabetes- and heart-friendly. Each recipe is designed to be easy to prepare, nutrient-dense, and satisfying for seniors managing osteoporosis.

Healthy snack recipes:

Almond Chia Pudding

Ingredients:

- 1/4 cup chia seeds

- 1 cup unsweetened almond milk (calcium-fortified)

- 1 teaspoon vanilla extract

- 1 tablespoon almond butter

- 1 tablespoon chopped almonds

Preparation:

1. In a bowl, combine chia seeds, almond milk, and vanilla extract. Stir well.

2. Let the mixture sit in the fridge for 2-3 hours (or overnight) to thicken.

3. Stir the pudding, then top with almond butter and chopped almonds before serving.

Number of servings: 2

Nutritional Information (per serving):

- Calories: 220

- Protein: 7g

- Fat: 14g

- Carbohydrates: 12g

- Calcium: 250mg

- Magnesium: 120mg

- Vitamin D: 100 IU

- Vitamin K: 3mcg

Cooking Time: 5 minutes prep + 3 hours chilling

Cucumber and Hummus Bites

Ingredients:

- 1 cucumber, sliced
- 1/4 cup hummus (store-bought or homemade)
- 1 tablespoon chia seeds
- 1 tablespoon sesame seeds (magnesium-rich)

Preparation:

1. Arrange cucumber slices on a plate.
2. Spread a small dollop of hummus on each cucumber slice.
3. Sprinkle chia seeds and sesame seeds on top before serving.

Number of servings: 2

Nutritional Information (per serving):

- Calories: 140
- Protein: 5g
- Fat: 8g
- Carbohydrates: 12g
- Calcium: 80mg
- Magnesium: 70mg
- Vitamin D: 0 IU
- Vitamin K: 15mcg

Cooking Time: 10 minutes

Baked Kale Chips

Ingredients:

- 2 cups kale leaves, torn into pieces (vitamin K-rich)
- 1 tablespoon olive oil
- 1/2 teaspoon sea salt
- 1/2 teaspoon garlic powder

Preparation:

1. Preheat the oven to 350°F (175°C).
2. Toss the kale leaves with olive oil, salt, and garlic powder.
3. Spread the kale in a single layer on a baking sheet.
4. Bake for 10-15 minutes until crispy, turning halfway through.

Number of servings: 2

Nutritional Information (per serving):

- Calories: 100
- Protein: 3g
- Fat: 7g
- Carbohydrates: 6g
- Calcium: 150mg
- Magnesium: 40mg
- Vitamin D: 0 IU
- Vitamin K: 300mcg

Cooking Time: 15 minutes

Greek Yogurt with Berries and Flaxseeds

Ingredients:

- 1/2 cup plain Greek yogurt (calcium-rich)

- 1/4 cup mixed berries (blueberries, strawberries)

- 1 tablespoon ground flaxseeds (magnesium-rich)

- 1 teaspoon honey (optional)

Preparation:

1. Spoon the Greek yogurt into a bowl.

2. Top with mixed berries and sprinkle with flaxseeds.

3. Drizzle with honey if desired and serve immediately.

Number of servings: 1

Nutritional Information (per serving):

- Calories: 180

- Protein: 10g

- Fat: 6g

- Carbohydrates: 20g

- Calcium: 200mg

- Magnesium: 50mg

- Vitamin D: 40 IU

- Vitamin K: 5mcg

Cooking Time: 5 minutes

Avocado and Sardine Rice Cakes

Ingredients:

- 1/2 avocado, mashed
- 2 brown rice cakes (whole grain)
- 1 can sardines in water (drained)
- 1 tablespoon lemon juice
- Salt and pepper to taste

Preparation:

1. Spread the mashed avocado evenly over the rice cakes.
2. Top each rice cake with sardines.
3. Drizzle with lemon juice, season with salt and pepper, and serve.

Number of servings: 1

Nutritional Information (per serving):

- Calories: 280
- Protein: 18g
- Fat: 16g
- Carbohydrates: 18g
- Calcium: 150mg
- Magnesium: 50mg
- Vitamin D: 200 IU
- Vitamin K: 15mcg

Cooking Time: 5 minutes

Cottage Cheese with Pineapple and Chia Seeds

Number of servings: 1

Ingredients:

- 1/2 cup low-fat cottage cheese (calcium-rich)

- 1/4 cup fresh pineapple, diced

- 1 tablespoon chia seeds (magnesium-rich)

Preparation:

1. Place cottage cheese in a bowl.

2. Top with diced pineapple and sprinkle chia seeds on top.

3. Serve immediately or chilled.

Nutritional Information (per serving):

- Calories: 180

- Protein: 12g

- Fat: 7g

- Carbohydrates: 14g

- Calcium: 200mg

- Magnesium: 60mg

- Vitamin D: 40 IU

- Vitamin K: 4mcg

Cooking Time: 5 minutes

Spinach and Feta Stuffed Mushrooms

Ingredients:

- 6 large button mushrooms

- 1/2 cup spinach, finely chopped (vitamin K-rich)

- 2 tablespoons feta cheese (calcium-rich)

- 1 tablespoon olive oil

- Salt and pepper to taste

Preparation:

1. Preheat oven to 375°F (190°C).

2. Remove the stems from the mushrooms and hollow them out.

3. In a skillet, sauté spinach in olive oil until wilted. Mix with feta cheese.

4. Stuff each mushroom with the spinach-feta mixture.

5. Place on a baking sheet and bake for 10-12 minutes until mushrooms are tender.

Number of servings: 2

Nutritional Information (per serving):

- Calories: 160

- Protein: 6g

- Fat: 12g

- Carbohydrates: 6g

- Calcium: 150mg

- Magnesium: 40mg

- Vitamin D: 0 IU

- Vitamin K: 200mcg

Cooking Time: 15 minutes

Walnut and Date Energy Bites

Ingredients:

- 1/2 cup walnuts (magnesium-rich)
- 1/4 cup pitted dates
- 1 tablespoon chia seeds
- 1 tablespoon unsweetened cocoa powder

Preparation:

1. In a food processor, pulse walnuts, dates, chia seeds, and cocoa powder until a sticky dough forms.
2. Roll the mixture into small bite-sized balls.
3. Store in the fridge for at least 30 minutes before serving.

Number of servings: 2

Nutritional Information (per serving):

- Calories: 180
- Protein: 4g
- Fat: 12g
- Carbohydrates: 16g
- Calcium: 50mg
- Magnesium: 70mg
- Vitamin D: 0 IU
- Vitamin K: 3mcg

Cooking Time: 10 minutes + 30 minutes chilling

Almond Butter and Apple Slices

Ingredients:

- 1 apple, sliced
- 2 tablespoons almond butter
- 1 tablespoon chia seeds (optional)

Preparation:

1. Arrange apple slices on a plate.
2. Spread almond butter on each slice.
3. Sprinkle chia seeds on top (optional) and serve.

Number of servings: 1

Nutritional Information (per serving):

- Calories: 220
- Protein: 5g
- Fat: 14g
- Carbohydrates: 24g
- Calcium: 60mg
- Magnesium: 80mg
- Vitamin D: 0 IU
- Vitamin K: 2mcg

Cooking Time: 5 minutes

Roasted Chickpeas with Garlic and Paprika

Ingredients:

- 1 cup canned chickpeas, rinsed and drained
- 1 tablespoon olive oil
- 1/2 teaspoon garlic powder
- 1/2 teaspoon paprika
- Salt to taste

Preparation:

1. Preheat oven to 400°F (200°C).

2. Toss chickpeas with olive oil, garlic powder, paprika, and salt.

3. Spread chickpeas on a baking sheet and roast for 20-25 minutes, shaking halfway through, until crispy.

4. Let cool and serve as a crunchy snack.

Number of servings: 2

Nutritional Information (per serving):

- Calories: 180
- Protein: 6g
- Fat: 8g
- Carbohydrates: 24g
- Calcium: 60mg
- Magnesium: 40mg
- Vitamin D: 0 IU
- Vitamin K: 8mcg

Cooking Time: 25 minutes

These osteoporosis-friendly snack recipes are easy to prepare, packed with essential nutrients for bone health, and designed to support overall wellness for seniors managing osteoporosis.

Delicious appetizer recipes:

Spinach and Feta Stuffed Mini Bell Peppers

Ingredients:

- 8 mini bell peppers, halved and seeded
- 1/2 cup spinach, finely chopped (vitamin K-rich)
- 1/4 cup feta cheese (calcium-rich)
- 1 tablespoon olive oil
- 1 garlic clove, minced
- Salt and pepper to taste

Preparation:

1. Preheat oven to 375°F (190°C).

2. In a skillet, sauté spinach and garlic in olive oil until wilted, then remove from heat.

3. Mix the sautéed spinach with feta cheese, salt, and pepper.

4. Stuff each bell pepper half with the spinach-feta mixture.

5. Bake for 12-15 minutes until peppers are tender and the filling is golden.

Number of servings: 4

Nutritional Information (per serving):

- Calories: 110
- Protein: 5g
- Fat: 8g
- Carbohydrates: 6g
- Calcium: 130mg
- Magnesium: 30mg
- Vitamin D: 20 IU
- Vitamin K: 150mcg

Cooking Time: 20 minutes

Broccoli and Cauliflower Bites with Yogurt Dip

Ingredients:

- 1 cup broccoli florets (vitamin K-rich)

- 1 cup cauliflower florets

- 1/4 cup Greek yogurt (calcium-rich)

- 1 tablespoon olive oil

- 1 garlic clove, minced

- 1 tablespoon lemon juice

- Salt and pepper to taste

Preparation:

1. Preheat oven to 375°F (190°C).

2. Toss the broccoli and cauliflower with olive oil, garlic, salt, and pepper. Spread on a baking sheet.

3. Roast for 15-20 minutes until golden.

4. In a bowl, mix Greek yogurt, lemon juice, and a pinch of salt to make the dip.

5. Serve the roasted broccoli and cauliflower with the yogurt dip.

Number of servings: 4

Nutritional Information (per serving):

- Calories: 100

- Protein: 4g

- Fat: 5g

- Carbohydrates: 10g

- Calcium: 90mg

- Magnesium: 30mg

- Vitamin D: 40 IU

- Vitamin K: 110mcg

Cooking Time: 20 minutes

Avocado Deviled Eggs

Ingredients:

- 4 hard-boiled eggs, halved
- 1/2 avocado, mashed
- 1 tablespoon Greek yogurt (calcium-rich)
- 1 teaspoon lemon juice
- 1/2 teaspoon paprika
- Salt and pepper to taste

Preparation:

1. Remove the yolks from the boiled eggs and mash them in a bowl with avocado, Greek yogurt, lemon juice, paprika, salt, and pepper.

2. Spoon the avocado mixture back into the egg whites.

3. Garnish with additional paprika and serve chilled.

Number of servings: 4

Nutritional Information (per serving):

- Calories: 140
- Protein: 8g
- Fat: 10g
- Carbohydrates: 2g
- Calcium: 50mg
- Magnesium: 15mg
- Vitamin D: 50 IU
- Vitamin K: 4mcg

Cooking Time: 10 minutes

Kale and Quinoa Patties

Ingredients:

- 1/2 cup cooked quinoa
- 1 cup kale, finely chopped (vitamin K-rich)
- 1 egg
- 1 tablespoon almond flour (calcium-rich)
- 1 garlic clove, minced
- 1 tablespoon olive oil
- Salt and pepper to taste

Preparation:

1. In a bowl, combine quinoa, kale, egg, almond flour, garlic, salt, and pepper.
2. Form small patties from the mixture.
3. Heat olive oil in a skillet over medium heat. Cook the patties for 3-4 minutes per side until golden brown.
4. Serve hot.

Number of servings: 4

Nutritional Information (per serving):

- Calories: 120
- Protein: 5g
- Fat: 6g
- Carbohydrates: 12g
- Calcium: 40mg
- Magnesium: 40mg
- Vitamin D: 20 IU
- Vitamin K: 130mcg

Cooking Time: 15 minutes

Cucumber and Smoked Salmon Rolls

Ingredients:

- 1 large cucumber, thinly sliced lengthwise

- 4 oz smoked salmon (vitamin D-rich)

- 2 tablespoons cream cheese (calcium-rich)

- 1 tablespoon chopped dill

- 1 teaspoon lemon juice

- Salt and pepper to taste

Preparation:

1. In a bowl, mix cream cheese, dill, lemon juice, salt, and pepper.

2. Spread the cream cheese mixture onto each cucumber slice.

3. Place a small piece of smoked salmon on top and roll up the cucumber slice.

4. Secure with a toothpick and serve.

Number of servings: 4

Nutritional Information (per serving):

- Calories: 120

- Protein: 8g

- Fat: 8g

- Carbohydrates: 4g

- Calcium: 40mg

- Magnesium: 20mg

- Vitamin D: 150 IU

- Vitamin K: 20mcg

Cooking Time: 10 minutes

Almond-Crusted Zucchini Fries

Ingredients:

- 2 medium zucchinis, sliced into fries
- 1/4 cup almond flour (calcium-rich)
- 1 egg, beaten
- 1 tablespoon olive oil
- 1 teaspoon paprika
- Salt and pepper to taste

Preparation:

1. Preheat oven to 400°F (200°C).
2. Dip zucchini slices into the beaten egg, then coat with almond flour mixed with paprika, salt, and pepper.
3. Place the zucchini fries on a baking sheet and drizzle with olive oil.
4. Bake for 20-25 minutes until golden and crispy.

Number of servings: 4

Nutritional Information (per serving):

- Calories: 110
- Protein: 4g
- Fat: 8g
- Carbohydrates: 6g
- Calcium: 30mg
- Magnesium: 35mg
- Vitamin D: 20 IU
- Vitamin K: 5mcg

Cooking Time: 25 minutes

Spinach and Ricotta Stuffed Mushrooms

Ingredients:

- 8 large button mushrooms, stems removed
- 1/2 cup spinach, finely chopped (vitamin K-rich)
- 1/4 cup ricotta cheese (calcium-rich)
- 1 garlic clove, minced
- 1 tablespoon olive oil
- Salt and pepper to taste

Preparation:

1. Preheat oven to 375°F (190°C).
2. Sauté spinach and garlic in olive oil until wilted, then mix with ricotta cheese, salt, and pepper.
3. Stuff each mushroom cap with the spinach-ricotta mixture.
4. Place mushrooms on a baking sheet and bake for 12-15 minutes until tender.

Number of servings: 4

Nutritional Information (per serving):

- Calories: 100
- Protein: 5g
- Fat: 7g
- Carbohydrates: 4g
- Calcium: 80mg
- Magnesium: 20mg
- Vitamin D: 0 IU
- Vitamin K: 150mcg

Cooking Time: 15 minutes

Walnut and Goat Cheese Stuffed Dates

Ingredients:

- 8 Medjool dates, pitted
- 2 tablespoons goat cheese (calcium-rich)
- 2 tablespoons chopped walnuts (magnesium-rich)
- 1 teaspoon honey (optional)

Preparation:

1. Stuff each date with a small amount of goat cheese.
2. Sprinkle chopped walnuts over the goat cheese.
3. Drizzle with honey (optional) and serve.

Number of servings: 4

Nutritional Information (per serving):

- Calories: 150
- Protein: 3g
- Fat: 7g
- Carbohydrates: 18g
- Calcium: 40mg
- Magnesium: 30mg
- Vitamin D: 0 IU
- Vitamin K: 2mcg

Cooking Time: 10 minutes

Roasted Red Pepper Hummus with Veggie Sticks

Ingredients:

- 1 cup canned chickpeas, drained and rinsed

- 1 roasted red bell pepper, peeled and chopped

- 2 tablespoons tahini

- 1 tablespoon lemon juice

- 1 garlic clove, minced

- 1 tablespoon olive oil

- 1/2 teaspoon paprika

- Salt and pepper to taste

- Carrot and cucumber sticks for dipping

Preparation:

1. In a food processor, blend chickpeas, roasted red pepper, tahini, lemon juice, garlic, olive oil, paprika, salt, and pepper until smooth.

2. Serve with carrot and cucumber sticks.

Number of servings: 4

Nutritional Information (per serving):

- Calories: 150

- Protein: 4g

- Fat: 8g

- Carbohydrates: 15g

- Calcium: 40mg

- Magnesium: 35mg

- Vitamin D: 0 IU

- Vitamin K: 2mcg

Cooking Time: 10 minutes

Crispy Parmesan Brussels Sprouts

Ingredients:

- 1 cup Brussels sprouts, halved (vitamin K-rich)
- 1/4 cup grated Parmesan cheese (calcium-rich)
- 1 tablespoon olive oil
- 1 teaspoon garlic powder
- Salt and pepper to taste

Preparation:

1. Preheat oven to 400°F (200°C).
2. Toss Brussels sprouts with olive oil, garlic powder, salt, and pepper.
3. Spread Brussels sprouts on a baking sheet, sprinkle Parmesan cheese on top.
4. Roast for 20-25 minutes until crispy and golden.

Number of servings: 4

Nutritional Information (per serving):

- Calories: 110
- Protein: 5g
- Fat: 7g
- Carbohydrates: 6g
- Calcium: 120mg
- Magnesium: 30mg
- Vitamin D: 0 IU
- Vitamin K: 200mcg

Cooking Time: 25 minutes

These appetizers are designed to be nutrient-dense, osteoporosis-friendly, and suitable for seniors looking to support bone health. Each recipe is rich in calcium, magnesium, vitamin K, and low in sugar and fat, while being easy to prepare.

Tasty soup recipes:

Creamy Broccoli and Spinach Soup

Ingredients:

- 2 cups broccoli florets (vitamin K-rich)

- 1 cup spinach (vitamin K-rich)

- 1 small onion, diced

- 2 garlic cloves, minced

- 2 cups low-sodium vegetable broth

- 1/2 cup unsweetened almond milk (calcium-fortified)

- 1 tablespoon olive oil

- Salt and pepper to taste

Preparation:

1. Heat olive oil in a pot over medium heat. Add onion and garlic, sautéing until softened (about 5 minutes).

2. Add broccoli, spinach, and vegetable broth. Bring to a boil, then reduce to a simmer and cook for 10-12 minutes until vegetables are tender.

3. Blend the soup using an immersion blender or regular blender until smooth.

4. Stir in almond milk, season with salt and pepper, and simmer for 5 more minutes. Serve hot.

Number of servings: 4

Nutritional Information (per serving):

- Calories: 110

- Protein: 3g

- Fat: 7g

- Carbohydrates: 10g

- Calcium: 200mg

- Magnesium: 40mg

- Vitamin D: 100 IU

- Vitamin K: 250mcg

Cooking Time: 20 minutes

Carrot and Ginger Soup

Ingredients:

- 4 large carrots, chopped
- 1 small onion, diced
- 1 tablespoon fresh ginger, grated
- 1 tablespoon olive oil
- 2 cups low-sodium vegetable broth
- 1/2 cup unsweetened almond milk (calcium-fortified)
- Salt and pepper to taste

Preparation:

1. Heat olive oil in a large pot over medium heat. Add onion and ginger, sautéing until softened (about 5 minutes).

2. Add chopped carrots and vegetable broth. Bring to a boil, then reduce heat and simmer for 15-20 minutes until carrots are tender.

3. Blend the soup until smooth using an immersion blender or regular blender.

4. Stir in almond milk, season with salt and pepper, and heat through. Serve hot.

Number of servings: 4

Nutritional Information (per serving):

- Calories: 100
- Protein: 2g
- Fat: 5g
- Carbohydrates: 13g
- Calcium: 150mg
- Magnesium: 35mg
- Vitamin D: 100 IU
- Vitamin K: 15mcg

Cooking Time: 25 minutes

Butternut Squash and Lentil Soup

Ingredients:

- 2 cups butternut squash, peeled and cubed
- 1/2 cup red lentils
- 1 small onion, diced
- 2 garlic cloves, minced
- 1 tablespoon olive oil
- 3 cups low-sodium vegetable broth
- 1 teaspoon cumin
- Salt and pepper to taste

Preparation:

1. Heat olive oil in a large pot over medium heat. Add onion and garlic, cooking until softened (about 5 minutes).

2. Add butternut squash, lentils, cumin, and vegetable broth. Bring to a boil, then reduce to a simmer.

3. Cook for 20-25 minutes until the squash and lentils are soft.

4. Blend the soup until smooth. Season with salt and pepper, then serve hot.

Number of servings: 4

Nutritional Information (per serving):

- Calories: 180
- Protein: 6g
- Fat: 6g
- Carbohydrates: 28g
- Calcium: 80mg
- Magnesium: 45mg
- Vitamin D: 0 IU
- Vitamin K: 15mcg

Cooking Time: 30 minutes

Tomato and Basil Soup

Ingredients:

- 4 large ripe tomatoes, chopped
- 1 small onion, diced
- 2 garlic cloves, minced
- 1 tablespoon olive oil
- 1 cup fresh basil leaves (vitamin K-rich)
- 2 cups low-sodium vegetable broth
- 1/2 cup unsweetened almond milk (calcium-fortified)
- Salt and pepper to taste

Preparation:

1. Heat olive oil in a pot over medium heat. Add onion and garlic, cooking until softened (about 5 minutes).
2. Add chopped tomatoes, vegetable broth, and basil leaves. Bring to a boil, then reduce heat and simmer for 15 minutes.
3. Blend the soup until smooth. Stir in almond milk, season with salt and pepper, and heat through.
4. Serve hot and garnish with extra basil leaves.

Number of servings: 4

Nutritional Information (per serving):

- Calories: 120
- Protein: 3g
- Fat: 6g
- Carbohydrates: 16g
- Calcium: 180mg
- Magnesium: 30mg
- Vitamin D: 100 IU
- Vitamin K: 150mcg

Cooking Time: 20 minutes

Zucchini and Cauliflower Soup

Ingredients:

- 2 zucchinis, chopped
- 1 cup cauliflower florets
- 1 small onion, diced
- 1 garlic clove, minced
- 1 tablespoon olive oil
- 2 cups low-sodium vegetable broth
- 1/2 cup unsweetened almond milk (calcium-fortified)
- Salt and pepper to taste

Preparation:

1. Heat olive oil in a pot over medium heat. Add onion and garlic, cooking until softened (about 5 minutes).

2. Add zucchini, cauliflower, and vegetable broth. Bring to a boil, then reduce to a simmer.

3. Cook for 15-20 minutes until vegetables are tender.

4. Blend the soup until smooth. Stir in almond milk, season with salt and pepper, and serve hot.

Number of servings: 4

Nutritional Information (per serving):

- Calories: 110
- Protein: 3g
- Fat: 7g
- Carbohydrates: 12g
- Calcium: 160mg
- Magnesium: 40mg
- Vitamin D: 100 IU
- Vitamin K: 80mcg

Cooking Time: 25 minutes

Kale and White Bean Soup

Ingredients:

- 1 cup kale, chopped (vitamin K-rich)
- 1/2 cup canned white beans, drained and rinsed
- 1 small onion, diced
- 2 garlic cloves, minced
- 2 cups low-sodium vegetable broth
- 1 tablespoon olive oil
- Salt and pepper to taste

Preparation:

1. Heat olive oil in a pot over medium heat. Add onion and garlic, cooking until softened (about 5 minutes).

2. Add kale, white beans, and vegetable broth. Bring to a boil, then reduce heat and simmer for 10 minutes.

3. Blend the soup slightly if desired or leave it chunky. Season with salt and pepper.

4. Serve hot.

Number of servings: 4

Nutritional Information (per serving):

- Calories: 150
- Protein: 5g
- Fat: 7g
- Carbohydrates: 18g
- Calcium: 150mg
- Magnesium: 40mg
- Vitamin D: 0 IU
- Vitamin K: 250mcg

Cooking Time: 20 minutes

Sweet Potato and Carrot Soup

Ingredients:

- 2 medium sweet potatoes, peeled and cubed

- 2 large carrots, chopped

- 1 small onion, diced

- 2 garlic cloves, minced

- 2 cups low-sodium vegetable broth

- 1 tablespoon olive oil

- 1/2 teaspoon ground cumin

- Salt and pepper to taste

Preparation:

1. Heat olive oil in a large pot over medium heat. Add onion and garlic, sautéing until softened (about 5 minutes).

2. Add sweet potatoes, carrots, cumin, and vegetable broth. Bring to a boil, then reduce heat and simmer for 20 minutes until the vegetables are soft.

3. Blend the soup until smooth. Season with salt and pepper, then serve hot.

Number of servings: 4

Nutritional Information (per serving):

- Calories: 160

- Protein: 3g

- Fat: 5g

- Carbohydrates: 28g

- Calcium: 60mg

- Magnesium: 35mg

- Vitamin D: 0 IU

- Vitamin K: 10mcg

Cooking Time: 25 minutes

Cabbage and Mushroom Soup

Ingredients:

- 2 cups cabbage, shredded (vitamin K-rich)

- 1 cup mushrooms, sliced

- 1 small onion, diced

- 2 garlic cloves, minced

- 2 cups low-sodium vegetable broth

- 1 tablespoon olive oil

- Salt and pepper to taste

Preparation:

1. Heat olive oil in a pot over medium heat. Add onion and garlic, cooking until softened (about 5 minutes).

2. Add cabbage, mushrooms, and vegetable broth. Bring to a boil, then reduce heat and simmer for 15 minutes.

3. Season with salt and pepper and serve hot.

Number of servings: 4

Nutritional Information (per serving):

- Calories: 100

- Protein: 3g

- Fat: 5g

- Carbohydrates: 10g

- Calcium: 50mg

- Magnesium: 30mg

- Vitamin D: 50 IU

- Vitamin K: 150mcg

Cooking Time: 20 minutes

Leek and Potato Soup

Ingredients:

- 2 medium leeks, cleaned and chopped
- 2 medium potatoes, peeled and cubed
- 1 small onion, diced
- 2 garlic cloves, minced
- 2 cups low-sodium vegetable broth
- 1 tablespoon olive oil
- 1/2 cup unsweetened almond milk (calcium-fortified)
- Salt and pepper to taste

Preparation:

1. Heat olive oil in a large pot over medium heat. Add onion, garlic, and leeks, sautéing until softened (about 5 minutes).
2. Add potatoes and vegetable broth. Bring to a boil, then reduce heat and simmer for 15-20 minutes until potatoes are soft.
3. Blend the soup until smooth. Stir in almond milk, season with salt and pepper, and serve hot.

Number of servings: 4

Nutritional Information (per serving):

- Calories: 150
- Protein: 3g
- Fat: 6g
- Carbohydrates: 20g
- Calcium: 120mg
- Magnesium: 30mg
- Vitamin D: 100 IU
- Vitamin K: 30mcg

Cooking Time: 25 minutes

These osteoporosis-friendly soups are packed with essential nutrients and are easy to prepare, making them perfect for seniors managing osteoporosis. Each recipe emphasizes natural, nutrient-dense ingredients that promote bone health while being heart- and diabetes-friendly.

Nutritious juice recipes:

Kale and Pineapple Calcium Boost Juice

Ingredients:

- 1 cup kale leaves (vitamin K-rich)
- 1/2 cup fresh pineapple (calcium-rich)
- 1/2 cucumber
- 1/2 lemon, juiced
- 1/2 cup water

Preparation:

1. Wash the kale leaves, cucumber, and pineapple.
2. In a blender, combine the kale, pineapple, cucumber, lemon juice, and water.
3. Blend until smooth. Strain if desired, and serve immediately.

Number of servings: 2

Nutritional Information (per serving):

- Calories: 60
- Protein: 1g
- Fat: 0g
- Carbohydrates: 14g
- Calcium: 100mg
- Magnesium: 40mg
- Vitamin D: 0 IU
- Vitamin K: 200mcg

Cooking Time: 5 minutes

Spinach and Orange Sunshine Juice

Ingredients:

- 1 cup spinach (vitamin K-rich)
- 1 orange (calcium and vitamin C-rich)
- 1/4 cup fresh mint leaves
- 1/2 cup water
- Ice cubes (optional)

Preparation:

1. Peel the orange and wash the spinach and mint leaves.
2. Add all the ingredients to a blender and blend until smooth.
3. Strain if preferred. Serve over ice if desired.

Number of servings: 2

Nutritional Information (per serving):

- Calories: 70
- Protein: 2g
- Fat: 0g
- Carbohydrates: 15g
- Calcium: 80mg
- Magnesium: 35mg
- Vitamin D: 0 IU
- Vitamin K: 150mcg

Cooking Time: 5 minutes

Carrot and Ginger Osteoporosis Juice

Ingredients:

- 3 large carrots (magnesium-rich)

- 1/2 inch fresh ginger root

- 1 apple (low-sugar variety)

- 1/2 lemon, juiced

- 1/2 cup water

Preparation:

1. Wash the carrots, ginger, and apple.

2. Cut the ingredients into smaller pieces for blending.

3. Blend the carrots, ginger, apple, lemon juice, and water until smooth. Strain if desired.

4. Serve immediately.

Number of servings: 2

Nutritional Information (per serving):

- Calories: 90

- Protein: 1g

- Fat: 0g

- Carbohydrates: 22g

- Calcium: 40mg

- Magnesium: 20mg

- Vitamin D: 0 IU

- Vitamin K: 15mcg

Cooking Time: 5 minutes

Cucumber and Celery Bone Health Juice

Ingredients:

- 1 cucumber (hydrating and low-carb)
- 2 celery stalks (calcium-rich)
- 1/2 lemon, juiced
- 1/4 cup fresh parsley (vitamin K-rich)
- 1/2 cup water

Preparation:

1. Wash all the ingredients thoroughly.

2. Cut the cucumber and celery into pieces for blending.

3. Blend the cucumber, celery, lemon juice, parsley, and water until smooth.

4. Strain and serve immediately.

Number of servings: 2

Nutritional Information (per serving):

- Calories: 30
- Protein: 1g
- Fat: 0g
- Carbohydrates: 8g
- Calcium: 40mg
- Magnesium: 20mg
- Vitamin D: 0 IU
- Vitamin K: 150mcg

Cooking Time: 5 minutes

Beet and Berry Osteoporosis Juice

Ingredients:

- 1 small beetroot (calcium-rich)
- 1/2 cup blueberries (antioxidant-rich)
- 1/2 cup strawberries
- 1/2 lemon, juiced
- 1/2 cup water

Preparation:

1. Peel and chop the beetroot.
2. Wash the berries and lemon.
3. Add all the ingredients to a blender and blend until smooth.
4. Strain if desired and serve chilled.

Number of servings: 2

Nutritional Information (per serving):

- Calories: 90
- Protein: 2g
- Fat: 0g
- Carbohydrates: 22g
- Calcium: 60mg
- Magnesium: 25mg
- Vitamin D: 0 IU
- Vitamin K: 40mcg

Cooking Time: 5 minutes

Almond Milk and Spinach Green Juice

Ingredients:

- 1 cup unsweetened almond milk (calcium-fortified)
- 1/2 cup spinach (vitamin K-rich)
- 1/2 cucumber
- 1 tablespoon chia seeds (magnesium-rich)

Preparation:

1. Wash the spinach and cucumber.
2. Blend the almond milk, spinach, cucumber, and chia seeds until smooth.
3. Serve immediately for a creamy, nutritious juice.

Number of servings: 2

Nutritional Information (per serving):

- Calories: 90
- Protein: 3g
- Fat: 5g
- Carbohydrates: 8g
- Calcium: 300mg
- Magnesium: 60mg
- Vitamin D: 100 IU
- Vitamin K: 180mcg

Cooking Time: 5 minutes

Avocado and Coconut Hydration Juice

Ingredients:

- 1/2 avocado (calcium and magnesium-rich)
- 1 cup coconut water (electrolyte-rich)
- 1/2 cucumber
- 1/4 cup fresh mint leaves

Preparation:

1. Wash the cucumber and mint leaves.
2. Scoop the avocado flesh and blend it with the coconut water, cucumber, and mint until smooth.
3. Serve immediately.

Number of servings: 2

Nutritional Information (per serving):

- Calories: 120
- Protein: 1g
- Fat: 7g
- Carbohydrates: 14g
- Calcium: 50mg
- Magnesium: 60mg
- Vitamin D: 0 IU
- Vitamin K: 25mcg

Cooking Time: 5 minutes

Carrot and Kale Power Juice

Ingredients:

- 3 large carrots (magnesium-rich)
- 1/2 cup kale (vitamin K-rich)
- 1/2 apple
- 1/2 lemon, juiced
- 1/2 cup water

Preparation:

1. Wash and chop all the ingredients.
2. Blend the carrots, kale, apple, lemon juice, and water until smooth.
3. Strain if desired, and serve chilled.

Number of servings: 2

Nutritional Information (per serving):

- Calories: 80
- Protein: 2g
- Fat: 0g
- Carbohydrates: 20g
- Calcium: 90mg
- Magnesium: 30mg
- Vitamin D: 0 IU
- Vitamin K: 150mcg

Cooking Time: 5 minutes

Tomato and Cucumber Refreshing Juice

Ingredients:

- 2 medium tomatoes (vitamin C-rich)

- 1 cucumber

- 1/4 cup fresh parsley (vitamin K-rich)

- 1/2 lemon, juiced

- 1/2 cup water

Preparation:

1. Wash the tomatoes, cucumber, and parsley.

2. Chop the vegetables and parsley into small pieces.

3. Blend all ingredients with water until smooth.

4. Strain if desired, and serve chilled.

Number of servings: 2

Nutritional Information (per serving):

- Calories: 50

- Protein: 2g

- Fat: 0g

- Carbohydrates: 12g

- Calcium: 40mg

- Magnesium: 25mg

- Vitamin D: 0 IU

- Vitamin K: 180mcg

Cooking Time: 5 minutes

Celery and Green Apple Juice

Ingredients:

- 3 celery stalks (calcium-rich)

- 1 green apple (low-sugar variety)

- 1/4 cup fresh parsley (vitamin K-rich)

- 1/2 lemon, juiced

- 1/2 cup water

Preparation:

1. Wash the celery, apple, and parsley.

2. Cut the apple into pieces.

3. Blend all ingredients until smooth. Strain if desired, and serve chilled.

Number of servings: 2

Nutritional Information (per serving):

- Calories: 60

- Protein: 1g

- Fat: 0g

- Carbohydrates: 15g

- Calcium: 50mg

- Magnesium: 30mg

- Vitamin D: 0 IU

- Vitamin K: 160mcg

Cooking Time: 5 minutes

These juice recipes are easy to prepare, packed with nutrients, and designed to promote bone health, manage osteoporosis, and support overall wellness for seniors.

Wholesome salad recipes:

Spinach, Orange, and Almond Salad

Ingredients:

- 2 cups fresh spinach (vitamin K-rich)

- 1 orange, peeled and segmented (calcium-rich)

- 2 tablespoons sliced almonds (magnesium-rich)

- 1 tablespoon olive oil

- 1 tablespoon lemon juice

- Salt and pepper to taste

Preparation:

1. In a large bowl, toss the spinach, orange segments, and almonds.

2. In a small bowl, whisk together olive oil, lemon juice, salt, and pepper.

3. Drizzle the dressing over the salad and toss gently before serving.

Number of servings: 2

Nutritional Information (per serving):

- Calories: 180

- Protein: 4g

- Fat: 11g

- Carbohydrates: 17g

- Calcium: 100mg

- Magnesium: 70mg

- Vitamin D: 0 IU

- Vitamin K: 200mcg

Cooking Time: 10 minutes

Kale and Quinoa Salad with Tahini Dressing

Ingredients:

- 2 cups kale, chopped (vitamin K-rich)

- 1/2 cup cooked quinoa (magnesium-rich)

- 1/4 cup cherry tomatoes, halved

- 2 tablespoons tahini

- 1 tablespoon lemon juice

- 1 tablespoon water

- Salt and pepper to taste

Preparation:

1. In a large bowl, combine kale, cooked quinoa, and cherry tomatoes.

2. In a small bowl, whisk together tahini, lemon juice, water, salt, and pepper to make the dressing.

3. Drizzle the dressing over the salad and toss well before serving.

Number of servings: 2

Nutritional Information (per serving):

- Calories: 220

- Protein: 7g

- Fat: 10g

- Carbohydrates: 25g

- Calcium: 130mg

- Magnesium: 90mg

- Vitamin D: 0 IU

- Vitamin K: 250mcg

Cooking Time: 15 minutes

Arugula, Walnut, and Pear Salad

Ingredients:

- 2 cups arugula (vitamin K-rich)

- 1/2 pear, thinly sliced

- 2 tablespoons walnuts (magnesium-rich)

- 1 tablespoon olive oil

- 1 tablespoon balsamic vinegar

- Salt and pepper to taste

Preparation:

1. In a large bowl, combine arugula, pear slices, and walnuts.

2. In a small bowl, whisk together olive oil, balsamic vinegar, salt, and pepper.

3. Drizzle the dressing over the salad and toss gently before serving.

Number of servings: 2

Nutritional Information (per serving):

- Calories: 190

- Protein: 3g

- Fat: 13g

- Carbohydrates: 18g

- Calcium: 60mg

- Magnesium: 45mg

- Vitamin D: 0 IU

- Vitamin K: 120mcg

Cooking Time: 10 minutes

Cucumber, Avocado, and Feta Salad

Ingredients:

- 1 cucumber, sliced

- 1/2 avocado, diced

- 2 tablespoons feta cheese (calcium-rich)

- 1 tablespoon olive oil

- 1 tablespoon lemon juice

- Salt and pepper to taste

Preparation:

1. In a bowl, combine cucumber slices, diced avocado, and feta cheese.

2. In a small bowl, whisk together olive oil, lemon juice, salt, and pepper.

3. Drizzle the dressing over the salad and serve immediately.

Number of servings: 2

Nutritional Information (per serving):

- Calories: 220

- Protein: 4g

- Fat: 18g

- Carbohydrates: 10g

- Calcium: 120mg

- Magnesium: 40mg

- Vitamin D: 0 IU

- Vitamin K: 30mcg

Cooking Time: 10 minutes

Broccoli and Chickpea Salad

Ingredients:

- 1 cup steamed broccoli florets (calcium-rich)

- 1/2 cup cooked chickpeas (magnesium-rich)

- 1/4 cup red bell pepper, diced

- 1 tablespoon olive oil

- 1 tablespoon apple cider vinegar

- 1/2 teaspoon Dijon mustard

- Salt and pepper to taste

Preparation:

1. In a large bowl, combine steamed broccoli, chickpeas, and red bell pepper.

2. In a small bowl, whisk together olive oil, apple cider vinegar, Dijon mustard, salt, and pepper.

3. Drizzle the dressing over the salad, toss, and serve.

Number of servings: 2

Nutritional Information (per serving):

- Calories: 200

- Protein: 6g

- Fat: 9g

- Carbohydrates: 24g

- Calcium: 100mg

- Magnesium: 70mg

- Vitamin D: 0 IU

- Vitamin K: 140mcg

Cooking Time: 15 minutes

Spinach, Strawberry, and Almond Salad

Ingredients:

- 2 cups fresh spinach (vitamin K-rich)

- 1/2 cup sliced strawberries

- 2 tablespoons sliced almonds (magnesium-rich)

- 1 tablespoon olive oil

- 1 tablespoon balsamic vinegar

- Salt and pepper to taste

Preparation:

1. In a large bowl, toss spinach, sliced strawberries, and almonds.

2. In a small bowl, whisk together olive oil, balsamic vinegar, salt, and pepper.

3. Drizzle the dressing over the salad and serve immediately.

Number of servings: 2

Nutritional Information (per serving):

- Calories: 160

- Protein: 4g

- Fat: 11g

- Carbohydrates: 14g

- Calcium: 80mg

- Magnesium: 60mg

- Vitamin D: 0 IU

- Vitamin K: 200mcg

Cooking Time: 10 minutes

Cabbage and Apple Slaw

Ingredients:

- 1 cup shredded green cabbage (vitamin K-rich)
- 1/2 apple, thinly sliced
- 1 tablespoon apple cider vinegar
- 1 tablespoon olive oil
- 1 teaspoon honey (optional)
- Salt and pepper to taste

Preparation:

1. In a large bowl, combine shredded cabbage and apple slices.
2. In a small bowl, whisk together apple cider vinegar, olive oil, honey (optional), salt, and pepper.
3. Drizzle the dressing over the slaw and toss before serving.

Number of servings: 2

Nutritional Information (per serving):

- Calories: 100
- Protein: 1g
- Fat: 7g
- Carbohydrates: 12g
- Calcium: 50mg
- Magnesium: 25mg
- Vitamin D: 0 IU
- Vitamin K: 120mcg

Cooking Time: 10 minutes

Romaine, Avocado, and Pumpkin Seed Salad

Ingredients:

- 2 cups romaine lettuce, chopped (vitamin K-rich)

- 1/2 avocado, diced

- 2 tablespoons pumpkin seeds (magnesium-rich)

- 1 tablespoon olive oil

- 1 tablespoon lemon juice

- Salt and pepper to taste

Preparation:

1. In a large bowl, combine romaine lettuce, diced avocado, and pumpkin seeds.

2. In a small bowl, whisk together olive oil, lemon juice, salt, and pepper.

3. Drizzle the dressing over the salad and serve immediately.

Number of servings: 2

Nutritional Information (per serving):

- Calories: 200

- Protein: 4g

- Fat: 17g

- Carbohydrates: 10g

- Calcium: 50mg

- Magnesium: 70mg

- Vitamin D: 0 IU

- Vitamin K: 90mcg

Cooking Time: 10 minutes

Beet and Goat Cheese Salad

Ingredients:

- 1 cup cooked beets, diced (magnesium-rich)
- 2 tablespoons goat cheese (calcium-rich)
- 1 tablespoon chopped walnuts (magnesium-rich)
- 1 tablespoon olive oil
- 1 tablespoon balsamic vinegar
- Salt and pepper to taste

Preparation:

1. In a bowl, combine diced beets, goat cheese, and walnuts.
2. In a small bowl, whisk together olive oil, balsamic vinegar, salt, and pepper.
3. Drizzle the dressing over the salad and toss gently before serving.

Number of servings: 2

Nutritional Information (per serving):

- Calories: 180
- Protein: 5g
- Fat: 11g
- Carbohydrates: 16g
- Calcium: 100mg
- Magnesium: 40mg
- Vitamin D: 0 IU
- Vitamin K: 30mcg

Cooking Time: 10 minutes

Cauliflower and Avocado Salad

Ingredients:

- 1 cup steamed cauliflower florets (calcium-rich)
- 1/2 avocado, diced
- 1 tablespoon chopped parsley (vitamin K-rich)
- 1 tablespoon olive oil
- 1 tablespoon lemon juice
- Salt and pepper to taste

Preparation:

1. In a large bowl, combine steamed cauliflower, diced avocado, and parsley.
2. In a small bowl, whisk together olive oil, lemon juice, salt, and pepper.
3. Drizzle the dressing over the salad and serve immediately.

Number of servings: 2

Nutritional Information (per serving):

- Calories: 170
- Protein: 3g
- Fat: 14g
- Carbohydrates: 10g
- Calcium: 50mg
- Magnesium: 35mg
- Vitamin D: 0 IU
- Vitamin K: 60mcg

Cooking Time: 15 minutes

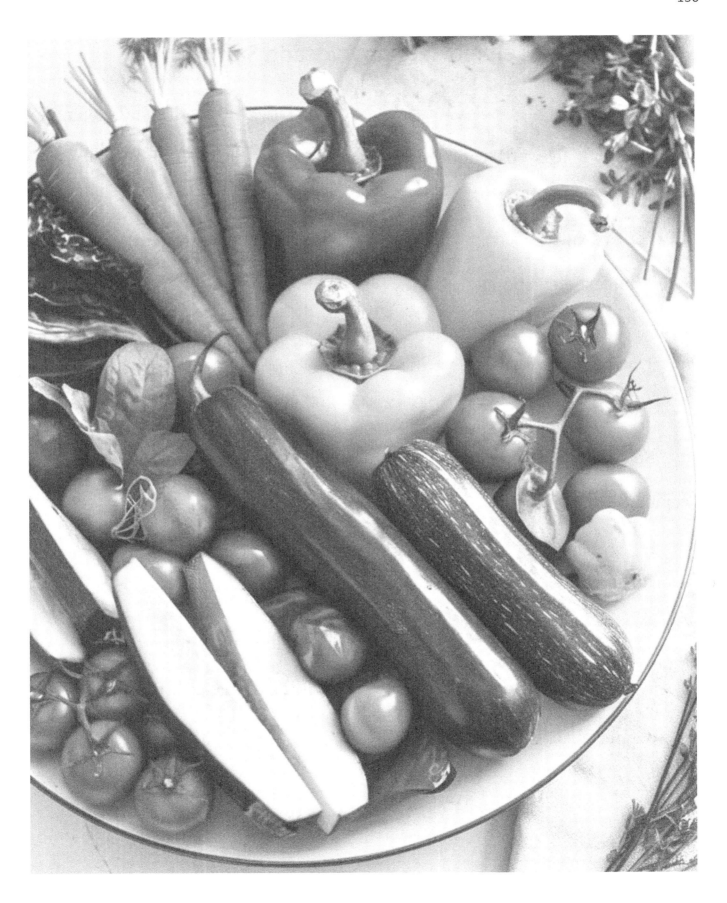

CONCLUSION

Osteoporosis can be a daunting challenge, especially for seniors, but it doesn't have to define your life. Through the pages of **The Osteoporosis Diet Cookbook for Seniors**, we've explored the power of food in not only managing but also reversing the effects of osteoporosis. By embracing a diet rich in calcium, magnesium, vitamin K, vitamin D, and other essential nutrients, you can take proactive steps toward strengthening your bones, improving your mobility, and enhancing your overall well-being. These recipes are crafted with care to provide maximum nourishment while keeping things simple and delicious.

Eating a balanced and nutrient-dense diet is not just about warding off osteoporosis; it's about living vibrantly, maintaining independence, and thriving in your golden years. With the right food choices, you can reduce the risk of fractures, improve joint health, and support your body's natural ability to rebuild and maintain strong bones.

The recipes in this cookbook have been designed with seniors in mind. They are easy to prepare, nutrient-packed, and tailored to your body's needs as you age. Every ingredient serves a purpose, from leafy greens and nuts that deliver high doses of vitamin K and magnesium, to fortified almond milk and yogurt providing essential calcium and vitamin D. Together, these nutrients work in harmony to keep your bones healthy and your body strong.

But the benefits of this diet go beyond physical health. Adopting a bone-friendly diet can also uplift your mental and emotional well-being. When you take control of your diet, you take control of your health. Each nourishing meal you prepare for yourself is a step toward a more empowered and fulfilling life, one where you can move freely, stay active, and enjoy every moment with confidence.

A Special Motivation

The time is now to make a change that truly matters.

By adopting the osteoporosis diet, you're not just committing to better health—you're investing in a future where you're stronger, more resilient, and full of vitality. Remember, it's never too late to start taking care of your bones. Every meal you enjoy from this cookbook is a celebration of the strength within you. You have the power to heal, to grow stronger, and to live each day to its fullest potential. Let food be your ally, and watch as your health transforms. Your bones will thank you, and so will your future self!

Bonus:

Creating an effective and simple 7-day exercise plan is essential for seniors who want to maintain strong and healthy bones. Weight-bearing exercises, balance training, and resistance exercises are particularly effective for increasing bone density and preventing osteoporosis. Below is a 7-day plan that includes exercises to strengthen bones, along with a step-by-step guide for each exercise.

Since I can't provide illustrations directly within this text, I'll describe the exercises in detail for easy understanding. You can find the illustrations online by searching the names of the exercises.

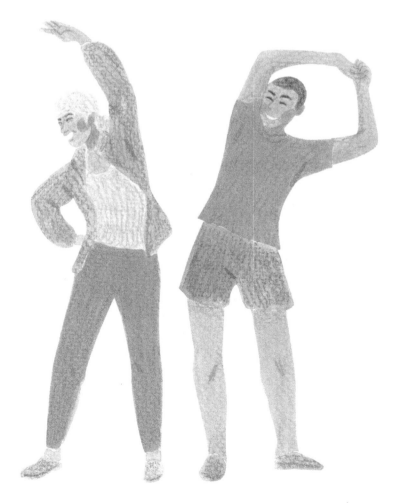

7-Day Exercise Plan for Strong and Healthy Bones

Day 1:

Walking and Standing Calf Raises

Walking (30 minutes)

- A low-impact, weight-bearing exercise that helps strengthen bones and improve cardiovascular health.

1. Walk at a comfortable pace in your neighborhood or on a treadmill.

2. Swing your arms naturally to engage more muscles.

3. Maintain a steady pace for 30 minutes.

Standing Calf Raises (3 sets of 10-15 reps)

- Targets the calves and strengthens the bones in your legs.

1. Stand tall with your feet hip-width apart, near a chair or wall for balance.

2. Slowly raise your heels off the ground, coming onto the balls of your feet.

3. Lower your heels back down to the ground.

4. Repeat for the recommended number of reps.

Day 2:

Bodyweight Squats and Plank

Bodyweight Squats (3 sets of 10-12 reps)

- Strengthens the hips, thighs, and lower back, which helps increase bone density in the lower body.

1. Stand with your feet shoulder-width apart.

2. Lower your body as if you are sitting back into a chair, keeping your back straight and knees behind your toes.

3. Push through your heels to return to a standing position.

4. Repeat for the recommended number of reps.

Plank (Hold for 15-30 seconds, 3 sets)

- Engages the core and strengthens your bones and muscles in the spine.

1. Begin by lying on your stomach.

2. Lift your body onto your forearms and toes, keeping your body straight.

3. Hold this position without letting your hips sag or lift.

4. Rest and repeat for the recommended time.

Day 3:

Yoga and Stretching

Chair Pose (3 sets of 10 seconds)

- Strengthens the legs, hips, and lower back.

1. Stand with your feet together, arms raised overhead.

2. Bend your knees as if sitting back in a chair, keeping your back straight.

3. Hold for 10 seconds, then stand up straight.

4. Repeat for the recommended number of sets.

Seated Forward Bend (Hold for 20-30 seconds)

- Stretches the hamstrings and lower back.

1. Sit on the floor with your legs extended in front of you.

2. Reach toward your toes, bending at the waist.

3. Hold the stretch for the recommended time.

Day 4:

Strength Training with Resistance Bands

Resistance Band Rows (3 sets of 10-12 reps)

- Strengthens the back, shoulders, and arms.

1. Sit or stand with your feet shoulder-width apart.

2. Hold the resistance band in both hands with the band looped around a sturdy object (like a chair or door).

3. Pull the band towards your chest, squeezing your shoulder blades together.

4. Slowly release and repeat for the recommended reps.

Lateral Leg Raises (3 sets of 10-12 reps each leg)

- Strengthens the hips and outer thighs.

1. Stand next to a wall or chair for balance.

2. Lift one leg to the side, keeping your knee straight.

3. Lower it back down slowly and repeat.

4. Switch legs after completing the reps on one side.

Day 5:

Balance and Core Exercises

Single-Leg Stands (Hold for 20-30 seconds, 3 sets per leg)

- Improves balance and strengthens the bones in the legs.

1. Stand near a wall or chair for support.

2. Lift one leg off the floor and hold the position, maintaining your balance.

3. Switch legs after holding for the recommended time.

Bird Dog (3 sets of 10 reps per side)

- Strengthens the lower back and improves balance.

1. Start on your hands and knees in a tabletop position.

2. Extend one arm forward and the opposite leg straight back.

3. Hold for a second, then return to the starting position.

4. Switch sides and repeat.

Day 6:

Light Jogging or Brisk Walking and Push-Ups

Brisk Walking (20-30 minutes)

- A weight-bearing exercise that helps improve bone density.

1. Walk at a faster pace than on Day 1, swinging your arms to engage more muscles.

2. Maintain a steady speed for 20-30 minutes.

Wall Push-Ups (3 sets of 10-15 reps)

- Strengthens the chest, shoulders, and arms, improving upper body bone strength.

1. Stand facing a wall with your arms extended at shoulder height, hands on the wall.

2. Bend your elbows and lean toward the wall, keeping your body in a straight line.

3. Push back to the starting position.

4. Repeat for the recommended reps.

Day 7:

Stretching and Meditation

Hamstring Stretch (Hold for 20-30 seconds per leg)

- Stretches the back of the thighs, supporting flexibility in the lower body.

1. Sit on the floor with one leg extended and the other bent inward.

2. Reach for your toes on the extended leg and hold for the recommended time.

3. Switch legs and repeat.

Cat-Cow Pose (10 slow repetitions)

- Stretches the spine and improves flexibility.

1. Start on your hands and knees in a tabletop position.

2. Arch your back (cat pose) while pulling your belly button towards your spine.

3. Then, lower your belly and lift your head and tailbone (cow pose).

4. Alternate between the two poses slowly.

Special Motivation to Adopt This Plan:

By committing to this 7-day exercise plan, you are not only increasing your bone strength but also supporting your overall health and mobility. Regular exercise has a profound impact on your quality of life. These simple, effective exercises help build bone density, reduce the risk of fractures, and maintain strong muscles. With dedication and persistence, you'll notice improvements in your balance, flexibility, and strength—leading to more confidence in everyday activities.

Your journey to stronger bones starts now. Let's get moving!

WEEKLY MEAL PLANNER

My Meal Planner

WEEK OF: _____   MONTH: _____

	BREAKFAST	LUNCH	DINNER	SNACKS
MON				
TUE				
WED				
THU				
FRI				
SAT				
SUN				

My Meal Planner

WEEK OF: _____   MONTH: _____

	BREAKFAST	LUNCH	DINNER	SNACKS
MON				
TUE				
WED				
THU				
FRI				
SAT				
SUN				

My Meal Planner

WEEK OF: _____   **MONTH:** _____

	BREAKFAST	LUNCH	DINNER	SNACKS
MON				
TUE				
WED				
THU				
FRI				
SAT				
SUN				

My Meal Planner

WEEK OF: _____   MONTH: _____

	BREAKFAST	LUNCH	DINNER	SNACKS
MON				
TUE				
WED				
THU				
FRI				
SAT				
SUN				

My Meal Planner

WEEK OF: _____   MONTH: _____

	BREAKFAST	LUNCH	DINNER	SNACKS
MON				
TUE				
WED				
THU				
FRI				
SAT				
SUN				

My Meal Planner

WEEK OF: _____   MONTH: _____

	BREAKFAST	LUNCH	DINNER	SNACKS
MON				
TUE				
WED				
THU				
FRI				
SAT				
SUN				

My Meal Planner

WEEK OF: _____   MONTH: _____

	BREAKFAST	LUNCH	DINNER	SNACKS
MON				
TUE				
WED				
THU				
FRI				
SAT				
SUN				

My Meal Planner

WEEK OF: _____   MONTH: _____

	BREAKFAST	LUNCH	DINNER	SNACKS
MON				
TUE				
WED				
THU				
FRI				
SAT				
SUN				

My Meal Planner

WEEK OF: _____   MONTH: _____

	BREAKFAST	LUNCH	DINNER	SNACKS
MON				
TUE				
WED				
THU				
FRI				
SAT				
SUN				

My Meal Planner

WEEK OF: _____   MONTH: _____

	BREAKFAST	LUNCH	DINNER	SNACKS
MON				
TUE				
WED				
THU				
FRI				
SAT				
SUN				

My Meal Planner

WEEK OF: _____   MONTH: _____

	BREAKFAST	LUNCH	DINNER	SNACKS
MON				
TUE				
WED				
THU				
FRI				
SAT				
SUN				

My Meal Planner

WEEK OF: _____   MONTH: _____

	BREAKFAST	LUNCH	DINNER	SNACKS
MON				
TUE				
WED				
THU				
FRI				
SAT				
SUN				

My Meal Planner

WEEK OF: _____   MONTH: _____

	BREAKFAST	LUNCH	DINNER	SNACKS
MON				
TUE				
WED				
THU				
FRI				
SAT				
SUN				

Made in United States
Orlando, FL
31 May 2025